GERD Acid Reflux And Gastritis Cookbook

Charles Thompson

Copyright© 2020by Charles Thompson

All rights reserved. This document is geared towards providing exact and reliable information with regards to the topic and issue covered. The publication is sold with the idea that the publisher is not required to render accounting, officially permitted, or otherwise, qualified services. If advice is necessary, legal or professional, a practiced individual in the profession should be ordered. -From a Declaration of Principles which was accepted and approved equally by a Committee of the American Bar Association and a Committee of Publishers and Associations. In no way is it legal to reproduce, duplicate, or transmit any part of this document in either electronic means or in printed format. Recording of this publication is strictly prohibited and any storage of this document is not allowed unless with written permission from the publisher. All rights reserved. The information provided herein is stated to be truthful and consistent, in that any liability, in terms of inattention or otherwise, by any usage or abuse of any policies, processes, or directions contained within is the solitary and utter responsibility of the recipient reader. Under no circumstances will any legal responsibility or blame be held against the publisher for any reparation, damages, or monetary loss due to the information herein, either directly or indirectly. Respective authors own all copyrights not held by the publisher.

The information herein is offered for informational purposes solely, and is universal as so. The presentation of the information is without contract or any type of guarantee assurance. The trademarks that are used are without any consent, and the publication of the trademark is without permission or backing by the trademark owner. All trademarks and brands within this book are for clarifying purposes only and are the owned by the owners themselves, not affiliated with this document.

Contents

Acid Reflux Diet Cookbook 7
Introduction 7
Chapter 1: Gastric Acid Reflux 9
    Causes 10
    Symptoms 16
    Treatments 19
    Risks and Complications 22
Chapter 2: Prevention of Acid Reflux 23
    How Does Food Help? 24
    Lifestyle Changes 29
    Impact of Exercise 32
Chapter 3: Treatment & Complications 36
    Treatment of Acid Reflux 38
    Complications Due to Acid Reflux 40
Chapter 4: Recipes for Breakfast 42
Chapter 5: Snacks, appetizers and side dishes 62
Chapter 6: Soups and salads 82
Chapter 7: Single course 101
Chapter 8: Fish 120
Chapter 9: Dessert 143

Conclusion	159
Gastritis Diet Cookbook	161
Introduction	161
Chapter 1: What is Gastritis?	163
Symptoms	167
Complications	169
Chapter 2: Diagnosis and treatment	170
Diagnosis	170
Treatment	172
Chapter 3: Diet	177
What are the most relevant diet tips for gastritis?	177
Chapter 4: Breakfast	185
Chapter 5: Appetizers, side dishes and snack	204
Chapter 6: Fish and Seafood	222
Chapter 7: Meat	236
Chapter 8: Unique dishes	252
Chapter 9: Dessert	268
Conclusion	285
GERD Diet Cookbook	286
Introduction	286
Chapter 1: Gastro-Esophageal Reflux Disease	287
Causes	287
Symptoms	289

    Treatments 291

    Risks and complications 296

Chapter 2: Prevention from GERD 297

    Foods to eat and avoid 297

    Impact of Exercise 299

    Lifestyle changes 300

Stress and anxiety can affect the proper functioning of the digestive system. Anxiety and stress have effects that fall on the stomach. A stressed brain negatively affects the general function of the organism. 301

Chapter 3: Recipes for breakfast 302

Chapter 4: Recipes for starter 316

Chapter 5: First dishes 331

Chapter 6: Main courses 344

Chapter 7: Recipes for Side dish 360

Chapter 8: Recipes for dessert 373

Chapter 9: Drinks&Shakes 388

Conclusion 399

Acid Reflux Diet Cookbook

Introduction

Acid reflux is a common digestive condition that creates irritation, heartburn, and pain at the opening of the stomach as well as burning in the food canal. A person experiences this issue due to the reverse flow of the fluid and food from the stomach towards the throat. All over the world, people commonly face acid reflux and other related issues, which can be worse if not treated on time and properly. According to health consultants, the increased ratio of acid reflux issues is due to inappropriate food consumption, poor food options, lack of sleep, stressful mental conditions, and lack of physical activity in people's everyday routine. The digestive system is a sensitive part of the body and can be easily disturbed due to any physical exertion or mental restlessness. The continuous problem with gastric issues can influence a person's productivity and thinking ability. It can restrict a person's activities and can be the cause of severe ulcer or esophageal cancer as well. the best and most natural way to treat acid reflux and its complications is a change of lifestyle.

Following proper diet plans and implementing exercise routines can help a person to overcome the reflux and improve their digestive health. People with obesity, diabetes, or who have inflammation issues can easily be affected by acid reflux. According to doctors, it is recommended that to overcome and avoid the gastric acid reflux, a person should maintain a healthy weight and keep active for at least 30 to 40 minutes at a time on a regular basis. This book provides enough information about acid reflux, its causes, symptoms and treatment options. As well as for the reader, it has the information that reveals how lifestyle changes can improve a person's overall health and reduce the signs and complications of acid reflux. For those with diet concerns, we have included some healthy and delicious recipes for those who are living with acid reflux. This way, those struggling with this issue can still have or enjoy the delicious food. It has many other interesting and informative facts about acid reflux and how to treat this condition with natural, healthy food.

Chapter 1: Gastric Acid Reflux

The human body is a complex one that is crafted very well. Everything is connected to each other and all the organs or tissues are working in perfect synchronization. If one thing goes wrong, then it will put a direct effect on the rest of the body as well. Our stomach is one of the integral organs of the body that affects many other parts as well. If your stomach is not working as it should, then your skin will be dull, and you will have acne, scars, heartburn, bloating, pain and a feeling of unrest. Among all these things, you may feel acid reflux in the body.

Acid reflux is a condition of having a burning pain that is similar to heartburn in lower chest or sometimes your food pipe or throat as well. When the stomach acid flows upward to the food pipe, it causes the acidic feeling to the pipe and lower chest. Sometimes in severe conditions is can come up to the throat, cause severe pain, and make you uncomfortable.

It seems to be a commonly experienced feeling by a majority of people in their daily routine, sometimes once in a week and sometimes in every 15 to 20 days. A person is diagnosed with the gastric acid reflux when he or she is experiencing the feeling more than twice a week. In such conditions, it is necessary for the person to move forward and ask for medical help.

Causes

Before heading for a doctor, it is necessary to look into the causes of acid reflux. Whenever our body is not functioning properly or an organ is behaving differently, there are certain reasons behind that. It is important to identify these reasons and problems in the first place. When you know the causes, you will be able to move toward a better treatment and prevention system. Therefore, here we are, discussing some of the major causes that lead to acid reflux.

Hiatus or Hernia

One of the non-preventable causes of acid reflux is the Hiatus or Hernia. It is a condition when a hole occurs in diaphragm that leads to the upper part of the stomach to enter the chest cavity. This situation can cause the acid from stomach to reflux in the upper canal and cause the burning sensation in throat and chest section.

It is one of the critical conditions in overall human health, as the person will not be able to control the factor. Only a surgery and proper treatment to the hernia can help to avoid the gastric acid reflux in such conditions. There is a 100 percent chance of acid reflux in hernia patients, as both sections intersect one other in this situation.

Obesity

Another cause of gastric acid reflux is obesity. When there is a lack of weight management, then our body behaves differently. Weight that is above average has an intense reaction in the body. Organs start behaving differently and this can result in issues. Obesity is not a normal condition; in fact, it is connected to a number of health risks. Increased weight and body mass affect total body stamina, bone strength, heart performance, blood circulation, hormonal changes and organ activities.

Gastric acid reflux is one of the major outcomes that are related to obesity. The stomach is unable to digest all the food properly, and the acid release is an effort to deal with the excessive energy left in the body. It causes the outward flow of acid from the stomach. Moreover, obesity can affect the stomach size and its movement can trigger the condition of acid reflux.

Smoking

Smoking is one of the biggest causes of acid reflux. It is a known fact that cigarettes and cigars have acidic reactions in the body. Moreover, smoking affects the overall organ system composition as well. It can not only affect the lungs, but the stomach as well. In response to the smoke and all the chemicals in it, the acid in the stomach reaches the food canal in reverse. When the person inhales and exhales smoke, it can come up with fumes of acid from the stomach and can increase the risks and effects of gastric acid reflux.

Alcohol

Another major cause of acid reflux is the use of alcohol. Alcoholism is dangerous for a person's overall health. It affects the lifestyle and internal organs of the body. The consumption of alcohol is good if kept within a safe limit, but when there is excessive use, there will be problems. Acid reflux is one of the problems that are caused as a result of excessive alcohol consumption. The important thing is to keep the consumption of alcohol in normal routine and keep it limited for the safe use.

No or low physical activity

The food we eat is digested in our stomach and the process is triggered by two major things. One is acid, and the other is physical activity. If a person eats and has no or low physical activity, then there can be a chance of acid reflux. The stomach will produce acid in order to digest food, but the excessive amount of acid will produce a reflux in the food canal in the event of no activity. It is important to have a walk after a meal or exert your body physically to trigger the proper digestion of your food. It will help you to make things better and smooth as well. Physical activity will help you to make the better use of acid in the stomach and get it dissolved in the food. It will neutralize the acid in the digestion process and will get you all the necessary nutrients you need.

Multiple drugs and sedatives

Sometimes the sedative medications and anti-depressant drugs we take can cause acidity in the stomach. That acidity can lead to ultimate gastric acid reflux. It is necessary to have a safe and limited dosage of the drugs. The excessive use of medicine, especially without prescriptions, could affect your overall stomach functions.

Pregnancy

During pregnancy, there are numerous changes that occur. From mood swings to food options and psychological ideas to physical movements, everything changes. During this process, females have threats to face, many of them being critical health constraints. It can happen sometimes due to lack of care, vitamins, or excessive use of a specific product. There are sometimes the genetic reactions in the body as well. Acid reflux is something that is not inherited, but it can be caused by pregnancy and body changes. Your stomach may behave differently and you may not be getting as physical movement, so it can lead to a reflux situation.

Moreover, the vomiting and constant nausea caused by pregnancy can always trigger the gastric acid reflux. In this regard, the important thing is to monitor everything and then have essential solutions.

Poor dietary selection

Your food intake and dietary choices matter a lot when it comes to your overall health. Acid reflux can be triggered by poor dietary options. If you are consuming junk food, soft drinks, dried snacks, and fat rich food options then you may feel the hits of acid reflux. Such food options increase the acidity in the stomach and can result in issues.

Improper posture after meal

Acid reflux is not just caused by medical deficiencies and complications. In fact, it can come up as a reaction to bad posture . It is necessary to ensure the proper physical posture when having meal. Bending over your waist or lying on your back while eating or right after taking meal can result in acid reflux. It can be dangerous and build up the issue for more serious causes. It is necessary to watch out during your meal and pay attention to your movement routine in order to avoid such drastic outcomes from your activities.

Bedtime snacks

Bedtime snacking is one of the common habits that people have. It is a kind of regular routine for people in many cases. On the other hand, it is one of the critical causes of acid reflux. Eating food at bedtime does not allow it to digest properly, and the physical posture that often accompanies bedtime snacking can cause the stomach acids to reflux upwards.

Symptoms

Most people confuse gastric acid reflux with heartburn. Sometimes it is claimed that both are same and sometimes they are marked as different. Although there is a fine line difference between the two, it is necessary to underline the difference focusing on the symptoms of acid reflux. You can fight with a medical condition after knowing its causes and major symptoms. The symptoms are necessary for the better evaluation and diagnosis.

Acid reflux is one of the conditions that people do not take seriously in the beginning. Lately, when things are a bit out of control, they became concerned about the issue. In order to live healthily, the important thing is to keep the symptoms and all changes in the body under consideration. It is good to know the major symptoms and take note of these symptoms. Eventually, it will help in self and early diagnosis and then you can come up with the best of remedies and treatments. Here are a few major symptoms of gastric acid reflux to consider:

- Heartburn is one of the major symptoms of acid reflux. It is not the same thing, but the first step that leads to the condition. You can feel a discomfort or pain with a burning sensation in your abdomen and chest area that goes up to your throat.

- Bitter tasting in back side of mouth and throat is another symptom that is shows the bad stomach condition and acid reflux
- Burning sensation in the upper throat can be a reaction of acid reflux
- You can feel nausea and an ultimate feeling of throwing up the food you just had
- Continuous burping with a bad smell and acidic feeling
- Vomit can be bloody and painful in severe cases
- Acid reflux can cause black and bloody stools, accompanied by a burning sensation
- There can be difficult hiccups with a mixed feeling of pain and burning
- The immense reduction in weight can be observed without any reason
- Sore throat, dry cough, and wheezing can occur in initial and chronic stages of acid reflux
- There can be a feeling of unease in the throat, like food is stuck in the throat and will be out in no time
- Difficulty in swallowing food, with pain and burning
- Bad breath and dental erosion are other major symptoms of acid reflux

The condition of acid reflux not only affects the stomach and causes a burning sensation inside. In fact, it leads to some major outcomes. If there is not proper treatment of the condition, then results can be drastic. It can start as a simple problem of indigestion or acidity in the stomach that will lead to burping and even up resulting in bloody vomit, difficulty in swallowing and much more. It is necessary to identify these basic symptoms initially and take measures in order to resolve these issues quickly.

You can get to know more symptoms of acid reflux in certain cases. It is not necessary that everyone will face the same issues in the beginning. The person could have any of these or all of these symptoms from time to time. The best way is to be alert with the treatment, even if you are facing the initial or minor symptoms. Sometimes you may have these issues mixed with any other health condition, then make sure to discuss this with your physician in the first place.

Remember, bad smell and throat issues largely come from your stomach, and if these go unnoticed, then you may have to face the music. Note the symptoms and related symbols of the problem and consider these things in your daily routine for early diagnosis and control of the problem.

Treatments

Gastric acid reflux seems to be a common and normal issue. However, in extreme cases,, it can be lethal. If you are ignoring the condition and not concerned about getting treatment, you will still have to face the issues in the end. Whenever a person is suffering from the acid reflux, it is necessary to go for the treatment and remedies in the first place. Without a proper and organized treatment, it is not possible to recover from the condition, and it can cause issues in the long run. Here are some treatment options that one could consider.

Medications

During the initial stage when a person is facing issues with heartburn or acidity, there are certain medications to use to control these symptoms. It is necessary to use these medications after the proper consultation. Remember you may mix up heartburn and acid reflux with each other. Heartburn can be a condition in acid reflux, but it is not the acid reflux all the time.

Gaviscon is one of the famous and commonly used drugs to treat problems related to heartburn. It is one of the mild and effective sources that help to reduce the burning in the initial scale. If you have the severe case of acid reflux, then you will get the drugs in combination of famotidine, ranitidine, cimetidine, rebeprazole, omeprazole and others.

Make sure to consult a physician in severe cases for the medication prescription and keep up with regular checkups.

Surgery

When it is not possible to treat the condition of acid reflux using medications, then doctors have another option: surgery. To treat conditions, there are two types of surgeries depending on the condition and the patient's situation. In the first type of surgical procedure, there is a placement of a LINX device around and outside the lowered end of the esophagus or food pipe. The device is made of titanium wires that work as a barrier to fluid flowing outward from the stomach. The device helps patients to quit or reduce medication intake. Having the device after a surgery comes with a number of limitations. For example, the patient can never have MRI test later on. Moreover, it is necessary to check if the patient is allergic to any metal or not.

The second surgical procedure is the fundoplication that helps to reduce the acid reflux. In the procedure, an artificial valve is attached to the top of stomach that wraps the upper part of the stomach and reduces the chances of acid reflux. It can be a treatment for the hiatal hernia as well.

Both of these surgical procedures should be considered a last resort in the case of acid reflux. The first preference in every case is prevention using lifestyle changes, the second is medication with major lifestyle changes. In the end, if the condition is critical and patient needs ultimate help, then surgery is the option that doctors should eventually resort to.

Lifestyle

Along with the medication or surgery when you are suffering from acid reflux, then you need to make some essential lifestyle changes. Adopting some of the right habits and making a difference in your routine will help you to be good and better with the treatment. Here are the major changes you need to make in your daily routine:

- Take a light and spice free diet
- Eat healthy and fresh
- Eat in intervals
- Take your medications on time
- Do not wear tight clothes or belts
- Take your meals in intervals and in small portions
- Increase your physical activity to help your body consume energy and reduce weight if you are overweight

Risks and Complications

If there is a lack of concern towards the issue and you delay treatment, then it can lead to some drastic complications. They can seem to be minor issues, but can never be so reckless that you must face the critical music. Here are the complications you may have to face:

- The borderline of the esophagus can be damaged and inflamed, causing constant irritation, internal bleeding, and ulceration in some cases.
- There can be a non-stop burning and internal irritation that can affect the overall health and enhance psychological pressure as well.
- There can be scar development that will lead to difficult swallowing and food will not be able to travel down the esophagus
- The repeated exposure of the cells and tissues to the stomach acid can change their formation. It can damage the cell structure, causing them to be dead and potentially leading to cancer development.

It is necessary to focus on the problem in the first stage in order to help with the proper treatment. In case of permanent negligence, things can be difficult to control and will come up with some of the ultimately damaging results as a whole.

Chapter 2: Prevention of Acid Reflux

Prevention is better than treatment, as we all know. It is not just a phrase but in all matters, it is the ultimate solution and escape. No matter from what disease you are going through, you need to make sure that you will adopt some of the important preventions that will help you to live a healthy life.

In case of acid reflux, things are quite manageable and in your hand. There are certain preventions that help to keep your body in order. It is not something that is caused by any external virus or infection; it is all about the mismanagement in your daily routine. With a little management and care, you can stop or revert things in the initial stage. It is quite easy to follow the prevention guide for acid reflux.

What are some common preventions?

The preventions for acid reflux are more related to your food options than hygienic conditions. It is a kind of lifestyle problem that can occur and trigger to your mismanagement with food, posture, habits, and lifestyle as well. Therefore, it is necessary that you follow some safe lifestyle options in order to avoid further damage to your body.

Using the prevention options, you will be able to avoid the factors that can cause acid reflux, such as heartburn, obesity, depression, drugs, hernia and much more. In our body, everything is linked with each other and you have to make sure that your overall body is healthy. Overall health is something that can help you to be good in life and avoid all the serious threats and issues.

How Does Food Help?

All problems related to stomach are directly connected to food. The food or diet we use is one of the integral factors in our body. All the minerals and nutrients we get from our food helps us to grow. In case if we do not eat properly or have the right food that we need, it means we can have some deficiencies in the body as well. From the beginning of our lives, cycle doctors recommend having the best food and diet plan in general. There should be everything healthy and well-composed in terms of nutrition, so the body will not have any deficiencies at all.

We once took care of everything in the diet since the birth of a child. Other supplements for nutrition are for emergency use when only diet is not helping the situation. Therefore, in order to prevent acid reflux, we need to get help from food in the first place. It is one of the best resources that will help you throughout life to manage the symptoms of acid reflux. If you want to avoid acid reflux, food helps.

If you want to treat acid reflux during the initial stage, food helps. If you have undergone surgery and are trying to maintain your condition, food helps. In short, no matter what your condition is, food is the factor that actually helps you to keep things in control. The question is how it can help you and what you can get out of it.

In order to prevent acid reflux using food therapy, it is necessary to make a food selection that helps you in the following manner:

Reduce acidity

It is necessary to eat food that reduces acidity and that does not have an acidic nature. As such, you cannot take coffee, alcohol, citrus and other foods that increase the acidic ratio in stomach. By taking the food that reduces acidity and that is lighter in nature, this will help your stomach to be better and reduce its acidic fluency. Moreover, it will not let the acid to reflux in the food pipe or cause burning in the stomach.

Provide the best nutrients

When you are recovering from acid reflux, your stomach is weak and it affects your overall body as well. You need to choose the food options with the best nutrients. Make sure to eat healthy food enriched with calcium, magnesium and phosphorus. Fruits like bananas, apples and berries help to reduce acidity. Make sure to avoid the processed food with many spices that can kill the nutrients in the food.

Reduce inflammation

Inflammation or burning is primarily caused by the unlimited spices and sauces we use in our food. It is necessary to take mild spices and sauces in order to keep your dietary choices light. The food spices can increase the burning sensation and double up the inflammation as well. You need to pick up food options with minimum spices or no spices in certain conditions. Moreover, choose to have anti-inflammatory food options that will help you to reduce the overall inflammation in the organs and body.

Helps to repair organs

There are food options like meat, white meat, grains, and sprouts that are enriched with protein and have the nature to repair body cells internally. The continuous acid reflux in the body causes the organs and cells to become damaged at a large scale. You need some extra nutrients to ensure the proper recovery of these cells and to have better health overall. In this manner, you need to pick up the food options that help in cell repairing and that makes you feel better from the inside out. It will be an overall benefit for you. Keep the digestion process lighter

Some major issues with the acid reflux are with digestion. The acid in the stomach is produced to digest food when we eat so much acidic food that the acid's ratio gets higher and causes a reflux. In order to avoid such conditions, it is necessary to eat food that is lighter to digest. It will help the stomach to produce a lesser amount of acid and digest the food easily. Moreover, the food will not be acidic in nature so it will get mixed in the stomach acid and neutralize the overall equation. It is a little science but overall helps to avoid any critical condition that will make you suffer in future on a larger scale.

The best food options to reduce and prevent acid reflux

Not all healthy diet plans or food options are effective

enough to help you with the acid reflux prevention and treatment. You need to pick up the specific combinations and safe food options that help to reduce inflammation, burning and acidity. Moreover, you need to keep a balance between your food intake so things will be balanced and work appropriately. Here are some major food options that you can use to prevent acid reflux or to have a quick recovery from the problem:

- Fresh vegetables that are rich in nutrients and low in fat and sugar
- Ginger
- Non-citrus fruits like banana, guava, apple, kiwi and more
- Lean meat and sea food
- Healthy fats like coconut oil, organic butter and more
- Egg whites

All these foods are not acidic in nature and reduce fats from the body. It is a good option to treat these foods as a priority. They can help in prevention and quick recovery from the acid reflux at the beginning. On the other hand, it's important to take a healthy diet seriously so that you can help your body to increase immunity and fight back these issues and problems.

Lifestyle Changes

In order to prevent acid reflux and have a quick recovery, in addition to controlling your diet, you need to make some lifestyle changes. These changes help bring about quick and effective recovery as well as prevention from the problem. These changes not only help to avoid the acid reflux problem but to have a better life and avoid any further health constraints.

Eat healthy

In your lifestyle changes, the very first thing you need to do is to eat healthy food. Even if you are eating processed meals, refined sugar, and other things, then make sure to substitute them with healthier alternatives.

There should be an irregular pattern of the consumption of these food options. You need to make healthy food options your priority in order to avoid such issues and complications.

Plan your meals

Make sure to take your meals on time at specific intervals. Eating too much or having meals with long breaks in between can never be healthy. You need to feed your stomach with a small meal after a specific interval so there will be no acidity in there. The planned interval based meals will help you in the path toward safe digestion.

Get 8 hours of sleep

Sleep is important to let your food digest and your stomach to work efficiently. Make sure that you are taking healthy and good sleep for 8 hours each night. It should be a quality night of sleep for a continuous 8 hours, not in breaks or parts. In the case of a partial sleep cycle, you will feel more exhausted and drained in the end.

Manage your stress

Stress and anxiety can actually affect the digestion system of your stomach. It is not ideal for a healthy living if you keep stressing out your body. Make sure that you keep a balance between work life and leisure time in order to relax yourself and avoid any health complications. A stressful brain affects the overall body functions and can cause acid reflux.

Maintain a balance between food options

Lifestyle changes are not about quitting the food options and limiting yourself to a specific kind of diet. It is about balancing your food options. You need to keep the balance between the food options you want to have and that you can have. Make sure that you pick up the right options that will help you to maintain a good balance in your overall intake.

Do not sleep immediately after meals

It is not an ideal habit to sleep or lay down immediately after having a meal. In such conditions, it is not possible for the stomach to digest the food properly. It increases the chances of acid reflux and acidity in stomach to a maximum level.

Increase physical exertion

Laziness and being in one place for extended periods of time is one of the triggers for acid reflux. If you are not having good physical activity in your daily routine, that means you are not letting your energy get consumed. In such a situation, the stomach acid stays in the stomach and is not be able to dissolve properly. This can cause refluxes later on. With the help of physical exertion, you will be able to reduce your weight and the chances of acid reflux.

Impact of Exercise
In the prevention and basic treatment, along with food, lifestyle changes and exercise will have a great impact on your overall results. Exercise and good physical activity can help your body to avoid many complications. Exercise activates all your organs, muscles and tissues. It allows you to consume all the energy taken from the food. Moreover, the stomach will digest the food instantly and the acid will not stay in your stomach later on.

Lean muscles

By reducing the amount of fats you intake, you have more chances of living a healthy life. In order to be happy and stress free from any issues such as acid reflux, you need to have a healthy body. Regular exercise helps you to have the lean muscles that mean you will have less fats and other related problems.

It will also reduce the chances of acidity in your body and allow you to consume all the energy from the food you consume food. Eventually, you can avoid many of the issues and problems related to acid reflux and other related problems.

Better organ functioning

When our body is in a resting position, it is not possible for all the organs to work efficiently. In the rest position or daily normal routine, not all your organs get the pressure and involved in the physical exertion. It causes these organs to have fats and face issues that can lead to some complications like acid reflux. Our stomach causes acid reflux because our stomach does not get the real word to do because of our inactivity. With the help of continuous efforts and activity, things can be better and you can avoid such problems.

Weight reduction

Obesity is one of the causes that triggers acid reflux. Workout and exercise not only helps keep your body healthy, but helps to reduce weight as well. It melts down all the fat from the body and gives you all good muscles and only muscular weight. On the other hand, it will help you to get better in the overall health scale so that you can enjoy your life.

Reduced inflammation

Exercise helps to break and make muscles and cells as well. The exertion activates the repairing muscles in the body that helps to reduce the internal and external inflammation. The acid reflux causes worse inflammation internally and makes the person unrestful. Exercise helps to deal with this painful condition and triggers the body to repair cells and damaged organs.

Active mind and healthy body

Along with food management, a good exercise routine is a perfect combination for a healthy body and active mind. By working out, you will consume all the excessive energy from the your food. Moreover it will release the stress and tension you have. In the end, you can have an active and peaceful mind with a lighter body. With all the exertion, our brain releases the stress hormones and eliminates them from the body in many ways.

Chapter 3: Treatment & Complications

Gastric acid reflux is not a chronic disease and people usually feel reflux after having a certain food. It is normal in several cases and can be eliminated and reduced with certain medical or natural remedies. But if it is not treated well or a person is having some digestive system problem, the problem can be persistent and become worse. The chronic disease of acid reflux refers to gastroesophageal reflux diseases. It usually occurs when a person constantly feels acid or food between the canal tube that is linked between the stomach and throat. It is also known as heartburn and creates discomfort and other potential risks to a person's health. In this scenario, a person feels or experiences the undigested food or stomach content in the food tube and to the throat. It can damage the inner lining of the tube and of the stomach walls as well.

Acid reflux quickly influences the people having any other health complications. For example, it is common in those with both type 1 and type 2 diabetes. People with asthma may also suffer from acid reflux. Poor digestion problems or other stomach related diseases can also create acid reflux. The treatment of this problem is necessary to be done on time to overcome other health complications, and if not done, then this can cause multiple serious consequences.

According to research, it is shown that acid reflux can be due to improper food intake and consumption of too much fried food and carbonated drinks. This can weaken the power of the stomach to easily digest the food and it can become reactive towards it. Sometimes other health problems can be behind gastric acid reflux. But during the initial stages, with the little concentration of food intake and lifestyle changes, the problem can easily be treated and overcome before it becomes a significant problem.

Treatment of Acid Reflux

Due to poor lifestyle and unhealthy routine, this leads to different health problems, and acid reflux is one of them. Our lives are too much occupied, even that it is hard to find time to eat at the right time. This increases bad food choices and leads to inappropriate meal times. This increases the weight of a person and can lead to obesity. These activities directly impact your sleep and mind activity. When a person does not have a sound mind and feels restless, the digestive system is the most sensitive part of the whole body. This system feels the effects of the stress first.. This leads to inappropriate food digestion and increases acid reflux.

According to the doctors and health advisors, acid reflux is a treatable problem, and with some lifestyle changes, it can be overcome easily. In the treatment of acid reflux, the first thing that matters is diagnosis. In the first recommendation, food that is not allowed to consume includes: fried and fatty food items, processed and canned food, carbonated drinks, alcoholic drinks, citrus, and pepper. These foods can increase the heartburn and restless condition and can create irritation or damage.

Other than the food restriction, it is necessary to reduce the size of the meal that a person consumes in a day. A large meal size can fill the stomach and increase the reaction or irritation. But with smaller meal sizes, the stomach can have a large space and as a result, this reduces the refluxes. As well as it is necessary to take the last meal 3 hours before going to sleep, and do not consume food right before bedtime.

To neutralize the condition, keep your head parallel to the body when you are on the bed. It helps to control the flow of food or acid towards the food canal and offer relieve for heartburn at nighttime. Do not use a high pillow, because it puts exertion or pressure on the stomach and can create a restless condition.

With the lifestyle and dietary changes implemented, keep consulting the doctor and get medication as well. The medication can help to neutralize the impact and prevent the acid reflux from gaining a serious impact on your health.

Complications Due to Acid Reflux

Acid reflux is a digestive related problem that can be treated with the medication and a change in lifestyle. But if not treated properly and if the condition is allowed to go untreated for a long time, then it can affect the stomach and other body parts as well. It is reflux or backflow of stomach acid or food towards the food canal that creates heartburn. Due to the movement of the fluid in the throat, a person may experience irritation and dry cough as well. A person with gastric acid reflux usually feels the pain in the chest that feels like a heart pain, but it is actually due to the gas and the effect of reflux comes from the stomach. Sometimes the symptoms get worse if not treated on time. Acid reflux can damage the inner lining of the esophagus or can be a reason for bleeding as well. This complication can create a stomach ulcer or can be chronic with time. Due to untreated stomach acid reflux, it is also noticed that some people even face the chronic problem of narrowing of their esophagus lining. With time, it can be the cause of esophageal cancer as well. This severe complication cannot just affect the person's health but also can be the cause of limited activities or reduced productivity. In the worst scenario, these can be life-threatening as well. The best remedy to avoid such issues is to keep the focus on a small problem and get the proper treatment from the health advisor on time.

If you are at the initial stage or facing the acid reflux, then it is important to pay attention to your activities. With just small change in their diet and lifestyle, a person cannot just overcome the issue but also get the treatment they need on time. Even with natural food and home-based remedies, it is easy to treat and control acid reflux. All you need is to avoid the unhealthy or acidic food choices that increase the acidity in the stomach. Consume the food with minimum spices and salt that reduces the irritation. Also have small meal sizes throughout the day. Furthermore, we have some recipes that will help you to make delicious food that offers relief for acid reflux as well.

Chapter 4: Recipes for Breakfast

1) Crêpes of chickpea flour with cabbage and fermented cashew nuts

Ingredients:
For the crêpes:
- 280 g of chickpea flour
- 500 ml of warm water
- 40 g of extra virgin olive oil
- 4 g cumin seeds
- 4 g sage
- 8 g of whole salt
- 10 cabbage leaves.

For the cashew spread:
- 150 g raw cashews
- 20 g white miso
- 8 g lemon juice
- 10 g nutritional yeast
- 3 g of whole salt
- 3 g yellow mustard powder
- water q.s.

For the crêpes: with the help of a whisk, mix the chickpea flour, water, and 20 g of extra virgin olive oil. Leave to rest for at least 8 hours. Then pick up the dough and season it with a mix obtained by blending the cumin, sage, and salt.

Mix well. Heat a non-stick or iron pot well, pour a teaspoon of sunflower oil, and distribute it well over the entire surface. Pour a ladle of batter, cook it until it comes off, then turn it over and cook it on the other side as well. When it is ready, place it on absorbent food paper and proceed with the dough. Cut the cabbage leaves thin. Heat a wok-like pan with the remaining extra virgin olive oil. Sauté the cabbage for a few minutes, add salt and let the vegetation water evaporate and it will come out. Keep them aside. For the spread: soak the cashews for 12 hours at room temperature, changing the water at least a couple of times. After that, rinse them well and put them in a blender along with all the ingredients. Blend until the mixture is creamy and without lumps. Serve the crêpes with the cabbage, a few flakes of cashew spread, and grated black pepper.

2) Almond cookies

Ingredients:
- 400 g of peeled almonds
- 400 g of light brown sugar
- 100 g of powdered sugar
- 50 g of flour
- 2 egg whites
- 20 g of water
- 1 teaspoon of yeast

Finely chop the almonds with 350 g of brown sugar. In a saucepan, over low heat, dissolve 50 g of sugar in 20 g of water. When the syrup is ready, add it to the almond mixture and the yeast, flour, and 50 g of powdered sugar. The mixture obtained must rest at room temperature for at least 12 hours covered with a damp cloth. After 12 hours, whisk the egg whites with 50 g of powdered sugar and mix them with the almond mixture (they are gradually incorporated by mixing them from the bottom up). Work until it is soft and homogeneous. Obtain some loaves that you will cut into small pieces and to which you will give the shape of the almond. Bake in the oven at 110 ° for about ten minutes. Let cool before serving with a sprinkling of icing sugar. Store them in a tin box to keep them longer.

3) Chocolate, almond, nut and coconut cookies

Ingredients:
- 100 g of dark chocolate
- 50 g of shelled almonds
- 50 g of walnut kernels
- 30 g of shredded coconut
- 50 g of whole coconut sugar
- 1 egg white whipped until stiff
- the peel of 1 organic orange
- 1 pinch of salt

Put the diced chocolate and the other dry ingredients, including the orange peel, in the mixer. Blend everything for a few minutes until it is reduced to a powder. You will get a rather lumpy mixture. Meanwhile, whip the egg white until stiff and add it to the dough, mixing carefully. Using a spoon, form balls of the mixture and place them on a baking tray lined with parchment paper. Try to distance them from each other because they will widen during cooking. Bake the cookies at 150 ° for 25 minutes. Let them cool before removing them.

4) Stuffed chickpea flour pancakes

Ingredients:
- 3 heaping tablespoons of spelled flour
- 2 heaping tablespoons of corn starch
- 3 heaping tablespoons of chickpea flour
- 2 tablespoons of oil and 1 pinch of salt
- 1 pinch of nutmeg
- 300 ml of partially skimmed milk

For the stuffing
- 1 small thistle (about 200 g) already cleaned
- 1 slice of clean pumpkin
- ½ small leek
- 2 teaspoons of flour
- 2 teaspoons of lemon juice
- 4 tablespoons of oil and 1 pinch of salt

For the batter: dissolve the flour and starch in a little milk, then gradually pour the remaining liquid and oil, beating with a whisk. When the cream is thick and fluid, add the salt and nutmeg. Let it sit for 20-30 minutes. For the filling: blanch the thistle in 500 ml of water where you have diluted the lemon and flour. Wash the leek and slice it thinly. Sauté it in a pan with 1 tablespoon of oil and 3 of water for 4-5 minutes, then add the coarsely grated pumpkin and the shredded thistle. After another 4-5 minutes turn off the heat.

Mix the batter. Just grease a non-stick pan and pour a ladle of the mixture into a thin layer. Cook the crepes for a few minutes on both sides. Stuff them and close them in a bundle. Serve hot.

5) Buckwheat pancakes with nettle sauce

Ingredients:
- **250 g of buckwheat flour**
- **150 g of nettle tops**
- **400 ml of soy milk**
- **3 tablespoons of white flour**
- **oil**
- **salt**

Put the flour in a bowl with the water needed to have a semi-fluid batter. Add salt, stir and let it rest for 30 minutes. Wash the nettles and blanch them for 5 minutes in a little salted water. Remove them with a slotted spoon and set them aside. Measure out 100 ml of their liquid (save the rest for other preparations). First, toast the white flour in a saucepan; first, pour the hot nettle water and then, always stirring and, little by little, the previously heated milk. Let the sauce thicken over low heat, then add the coarsely chopped nettles. Season with salt and season with a tablespoon and a half of oil. Heat a little oil in a pan and cook a ladle of batter at a time until you have not too thin crepes. Serve with the nettle sauce.

6) Savory pie with red lentils

Ingredients:
For the base (pan diameter 24 cm)
- 250 g wholemeal flour
- 3 tablespoons of extra virgin olive oil
- a teaspoon of natural yeast
- a teaspoon of whole sea salt
- water q.s.

For the filling
- 3 medium potatoes
- 2 glasses of red lentils
- a clove of garlic
- a slice of ginger
- half a small pepper
- 2 sage leaves
- extra virgin olive oil as needed
- whole sea salt to taste
- water or vegetable broth to taste

To garnish the surface of the cake
- Sesame seeds
- poppy seeds
- chopped almonds to taste

In a large bowl, pour the flour, salt, and yeast and mix well. Make a hole in the center in which to put the oil and, a little at a time, the water needed to knead. Work vigorously until you have obtained a compact but soft, elastic, and not stiff dough. Let it rest for 30 minutes in the fridge. In a saucepan, boil some water with a handful of coarse salt and the unpeeled potatoes. Cook them until they are soft. Drain them, let them cool and peel them. With a puree or a fork, mash them well. Mix well and set aside. In the meantime, put a drizzle of oil in a saucepan, heat and fry the whole clove of crushed garlic and the chili pepper, add a little water, then add the finely chopped ginger, the sage, and the lentils previously washed under running water. Mix well and add the hot water or vegetable broth necessary to cover the lentils. Salt. Set aside more hot water or broth, which will be added during cooking. Usually, in 15-20 minutes, they are cooked, do not worry if they fall apart slightly. The flavor given to the cake does not vary. After cooking, let them cool. Roll out your base with the help of a rolling pin until you get an elastic dough, not too thin because it must support and give body to the cake.

Line a baking sheet with parchment paper and lay the base on top, cutting off the excess edge, which you can use to prepare decorative strips for the surface. After removing the garlic and sage leaves, add the lentils to the potatoes. Mix well, seasoning with salt. Place the filling on the base, pour over a cascade of sesame seeds, chopped almonds, and poppy seeds. If you want, lay the puff pastry strips on top of the cake, forming the characteristic grid. Add a drizzle of oil on the surface and bake at 200 ° for about 40 minutes. Let it cool down a bit before serving. This savory pie is excellent when accompanied by raw and cooked seasonal vegetables.

7) Savory pie with potatoes and creamy mushrooms

Ingredients:
- 250 g of wholemeal flour
- 3 tablespoons of sourdough
- soya milk
- 1 teaspoon of brown sugar
- 2 tablespoons of oil
- 6 medium potatoes
- 200 g of mushrooms
- 100 g of sour cream
- 150 g of ricotta
- 2 cloves of garlic
- 1 teaspoon of marjoram
- 2 teaspoons of sweet paprika
- sea salt

Mix the flour with the sourdough, a little salt, and the lukewarm milk necessary to have a firm and homogeneous dough. Knead it for a long time on a table, wrap it into a ball and let it rise in a warm place for 4-5 hours. Meanwhile, wash the potatoes and steam them with the peel. While these are getting warm, peel the mushrooms and stew them in a pan with minced garlic, paprika, marjoram, and a little salt. When soft, add the cream and crumbled goat cheese. Peel the potatoes and cut them into slices about 1 cm thick. Roll out two thirds of the dough and use it to line a floured, rectangular, or round, high mold. Spread the potatoes inside, cover with mushrooms. Roll out the rest of the dough so that it covers the entire surface. Seal the edges well, brush with a little warm milk and bake at 180 degrees for 30-35 minutes. Serve the cake hot.

8) Energy cookies with oats and raisins

Ingredients:
- 300 g of rolled oats
- 100 g of raisins
- the grated zest of a lemon
- the zest of a grated orange
- 150 g of rice malt
- a teaspoon of ground cinnamon
- a teaspoon of vanilla powder
- apple juice to taste

First, soak the raisins in warm water for about 15 minutes, turn on the oven at 180 ° and prepare a pan lined with parchment paper to lay the biscuits to cook them. Once this is done, you can dedicate yourself to the dough, starting with toasting the oat flakes in a hot pan for a few minutes, stirring often. Place them still hot in a large bowl in which you will add the grated citrus peel, cinnamon, vanilla powder, and finally, the well squeezed raisins. At this point, add the malt to the mixture; knead with your hands with the help of a little apple juice (just enough to be able to work the dough without making it too liquid). You can proceed by taking some of the dough to form balls that you will crush in your hands to give it the classic shape of a round biscuit.

During this step, you can help yourself by wetting your hands with water. Place each biscuit in the pan and bake for about 10-15 minutes. Remove the pan from the oven and let the cookies cool. When they are cold, you can store them in an airtight jar, where they will keep well for a whole week.

9) Soft fruit plumcake

Ingredients:
- 300 g of buckwheat flour
- 80 g of sugar
- 1 sachet of yeast
- 5 tablespoons of oil
- 2 egg whites
- the zest of 1 grated lemon
- 1 jar of low-fat yogurt
- 100 g of shelled walnuts
- fresh berries (blueberries, currants, raspberries)

Mix the flour, sugar, oil, and yeast in a bowl, stir in the yogurt and lemon zest. Separately, whisk the egg whites and add them gently to the previous ingredients.
Finally, mix the walnuts and berries into the mixture.
Line a loaf pan with baking paper and pour the mixture. Bake at 180 degrees for about 40 minutes. If you want, you can serve this dessert with more low-fat yogurt and some fresh fruit.

10) Omelette with potatoes

Ingredients:
- 800 g of potatoes
- 6 eggs
- 2 cloves of garlic
- 2 tablespoons of oil
- 1 pinch of nutmeg
- 1 pinch of parsley
- 1 pinch of chives
- pepper
- salt

Finely slice and garlic. Wash and peel the potatoes and cut them into cubes. Fry the garlic in a pan with olive oil and water, add the potatoes, and cook them until tender. Season with the chopped parsley and chives and mix well. Beat the eggs, add the grated nutmeg to taste, and pour the mixture over the potatoes. When the eggs have hardened, turn the omelette and finish cooking on the other side. Serve immediately.

11) Oat porridge with chocolate, cashew and orange

Ingredients:
- about 10 tablespoons of oat flakes
- a few pinches of ground cinnamon
- a few pinches of vanilla powder
- 2 tablespoons of rice syrup
- 6-7 cashews
- dark chocolate to taste
- almond milk
- a slice of orange

Put the oat flakes in a bowl, then pour enough milk to cover them abundantly. Let it rest in the fridge overnight. The next morning add the cinnamon, vanilla, rice syrup and mix well. Add more milk if necessary. Complete with crumbled or chopped cashews, dark chocolate into small pieces, and a slice of orange. Consume the porridge immediately.

12) Plum gluten-free muffins

Ingredients:
- 300 g of cooked prunes
- 4 eggs
- 150 g of brown sugar
- 190 g of potato starch
- 200 g of rice flour
- 1 vanilla pod

Whisk the whole eggs with the sugar and the seeds of the vanilla pod. Add the starch, flour, and plums with their liquid to the mixture. Mix well and arrange everything in lightly oiled cups or silicone muffin molds; you should get 7-10 muffins depending on the molds' size. Bake in the oven at 180-190 ° for about 25 minutes, or until it comes out dry by inserting a toothpick inside the cake.

13) Pear, chocolate and hazelnut muffins

Ingredients:
- 3 cups of kamut
- 2 tablespoons of cream of tartar
- half a teaspoon of ground cinnamon
- half a cup of toasted hazelnuts
- half a cup of dark chocolate
- half a cup of sunflower oil
- half a cup of wheat malt
- 1 and a half cups of soy milk
- 1 large cup of pears in small pieces
- 1 pinch of salt

Mix the flour, salt, cream of tartar, and cinnamon in a bowl; in another, emulsify the oil with the malt and milk, then pour it into the first, mixing everything without stirring much. Add the coarsely chopped hazelnuts and chocolate, the peeled and chopped pears. Spread the mixture into muffin cups and bake at 180 degrees for about 30 minutes.

Note: In this recipe, one cup is approximately 120 grams.

14) Pancakes without butter

Ingredients:
- Low-fat white yogurt 125 g
- 00 flour 150 g
- Skimmed milk 200 g
- Eggs 1
- Powdered yeast for cakes 8 g
- Extra virgin olive oil q.s.

Start by placing the egg in a bowl and beating it with a whisk. When it is light and fluffy, add the milk slowly and, continue to beat, add the yogurt. Then add, passing it through a sieve, the flour, and the baking powder. Proceed by mixing carefully, with gentle movements from the bottom to the top, to not disassemble the mixture, until you get a smooth and homogeneous batter. Cover with cling film, and place it in the fridge to rest for about 30 minutes. After this time, recover the batter and heat a non-stick pan with a drizzle of oil over medium heat. Pour a spoonful of batter into the center of the pan, letting it spread by itself. After a few minutes, when small bubbles begin to bloom on the surface, it is time to turn the pancake with the help of a spatula. So cook it for another minute and when it's ready, place it on a plate. Continue like this until the batter is used up. Serve your butter-free pancakes with honey!

15) Gluten free sponge cake

Ingredients:
- **Eggs 5**
- **Brown sugar 150 g**
- **Vanilla bean 1**
- **Corn starch gluten free 150 g**

Start by placing the eggs in a planetary mixer, then add the sugar and whisk the ingredients for at least 10/15 minutes with a whisk until the mixture is frothy, puffy, and light yellow. If you wish, when the mixture is well whipped, you can add the seeds of the vanilla pod that you have cut in half and continue whipping for a few seconds to mix it well and flavor the mixture. At this point, you can add the starch (or potato starch) that you have previously well sieved: mix everything with a wooden spoon until you get a homogeneous mixture, being careful not to dismantle it. Grease and flour a round pan with a diameter of 24 cm with the starch, pour the dough into the mold's center, leveling it well. Bake the gluten-free sponge cake for about 35-40 minutes at 180 ° C in a preheated static oven without ever opening the oven in the first half-hour of cooking. Remove the mold from the oven and let the sponge cake cool in the mold before opening it.

Chapter 5: Snacks, appetizers and side dishes

1) Brussels sprouts with pears and walnuts

Ingredients
- 350 g of Brussels sprouts
- 40 g of leek
- 1 small pear
- 60 g of shelled walnuts
- 2 juniper berries
- salt
- 4 tablespoons of oil

Clean and wash the vegetables. Remove the most damaged leaves from the sprouts and divide them into four wedges; add them to the finely sliced leek, which you will dry for 5 minutes in a pan with 2 tablespoons of oil, half a glass of water, and the juniper. Cut the pear into cubes and coarsely chop the walnuts; add them to the mixture and continue cooking for another 3 minutes. Before removing from the heat, season with salt, season with the remaining oil, and stir.

2) Slices of crispy bread with black cabbage and beans

Ingredients:
- **200 grams of dry beans**
- **300 grams of black cabbage**
- **10 slices of wholemeal bread**
- **7-8 cm of kombu seaweed**
- **a few sage leaves**
- **3 cloves of garlic**
- **extra virgin olive oil as needed**
- **Salt and Pepper To Taste**

Soak the beans overnight, remove the soaking water and cook them in plenty of cold water, with the kombu, sage and a clove of garlic, possibly in an earthenware pot, for about two hours or until tender. Low fire. Season with salt and pepper in the last 10 minutes of cooking; remove the kombu, sprinkle the beans with a drizzle of oil and set aside. Meanwhile, peel the black cabbage by removing the fibrous central rib, wash it well and cook the leaves immersed in lightly salted water, until tender (the black cabbage can be more or less tough). Drain, season with oil and a grind of pepper. Place the slices of bread in the oven and brown them on both sides. Rub them immediately with the remaining garlic. Place them on a serving dish and cover with the beans and black cabbage. Serve immediately.

3) Broccoli with miso sauce and nuts

Ingredients:
- 2-3 broccoli tops
- 80 g of walnuts
- 2 tablespoons of miso
- about 1 cm of ginger root

Cut and wash the broccoli tops and place them in the steamer basket, adding a pinch of salt. Cook in a covered pot until the broccoli is tender but still bright green. Meanwhile, toast the walnuts in the oven at 180° until they are fragrant. Let them cool down. Chop them coarsely by hand to prevent them from releasing too much oil, and then grind them in a mixer with miso and water or vegetable broth, just enough to obtain a smooth cream. Flavor with the ginger juice, obtained by squeezing the grated root. Serve the vegetables with the sauce.

4) Tofu with pear and spinach

Ingredients:
- 200 g of natural tofu
- 2-3 large handfuls of fresh spinach
- 1 ripe but firm pear
- ½ leek
- 3-4 tablespoons of oil
- 2-3 tablespoons of tamari
- lemon juice, to taste
- whole sea salt, to taste

Clean the vegetables and slice the leek into more or less thin slices. Wash the pear and cut it into pieces. In a heavy-bottomed pan, heat the oil over high heat, add the tamari, and let the leek dry. Also, add the tofu cut into cubes and let it brown on all sides, turning often. Remove from the heat and transfer the tofu with leeks to a salad bowl along with the cleaned spinach and pear slices. Season with the oil of olive to taste, lemon juice and salt, mix and serve.

5) Sweet and sour stewed pumpkin

Ingredients:
- **3 cups of chopped pumpkin**
- **2 tablespoons of extra virgin olive oil**
- **chopped sage to taste**
- **water q.s.**
- **2 tablespoons of rice vinegar**
- **salt**

Heat the oil in a pot with the chopped sage and rosemary, then add the pumpkin, a little salt and sauté for a few minutes. Add a little water and vinegar, cover, and let it simmer over low heat for about 15-20 minutes until the pumpkin is tender.

6) Sweet potato with coriander and curry with ginger and citrus sauce

Ingredients:
- 900 g of sweet potatoes
- 300 ml of vegetable cream
- lemon juice
- the grated zest of 1 lemon
- 6 cm of fresh ginger root
- 4-5 tablespoons of oil
- half a tablespoon of coriander powder
- half a tablespoon of curry powder
- sea salt to taste
- fresh parsley, to taste
- freshly ground black pepper, to taste

Preheat the oven to 180 degrees. Wash the potatoes well, but don't peel them. Cut them into wedges lengthwise and arrange them on a baking tray that you have lined with baking paper. Brush the potatoes with oil, season with coriander, curry, pepper, salt, and bake. Meanwhile, prepare the sauce by mixing the vegetable cream, lime juice, lemon zest, peeled and grated ginger, and salt in a bowl. Set the sauce aside. Remove the potatoes from the oven when they are tender and golden and serve with a little sauce and the freshly chopped parsley.

7) Quick pizzas

Ingredients:
For the dough
- 200 g of finely ground millet
- 200 g of rice flour
- 3 tablespoons of oil
- 1 teaspoon of salt
- 1 tablespoon yeast
- 1 tablespoon of sesame and flax seeds

For the filling:
- 500 g of clean pumpkin
- 1 sprig of sage
- 1 sprig of rosemary
- 2 tablespoons of oil

For the mini pizzas: Finely chop the seeds. Combine them with the other ingredients in a large bowl and knead with your hands to get a soft and homogeneous mixture. Let it rest for about 1 hour. For the filling. Cut the pumpkin into cubes, sprinkle with chopped sage and rosemary. Cook it in steam or the oven for 15-20 minutes, let it cool, and season with oil. Blend it until you have a cream, helping you if needed with a little water. Roll out the not too thin dough with a rolling pin and cut out discs with the help of a glass; place them on a baking sheet lined with parchment paper and cover with the cream. Bake at 170 degrees for about 15 minutes.

8) Mushrooms with orange spinach

Ingredients:
- 400 g of fresh spinach leaves
- 150 g of champignon mushrooms
- 2 large handfuls of shelled almonds
- the juice of 1 blond orange
- oil
- white pepper, to taste
- pink Himalayan salt, to taste

Clean the spinach and the mushrooms, which you will then have to slice thinly. Put the vegetables in a bowl with the peeled and chopped almonds and mix well. Season with orange juice, oil, a few pinches of Himalayan salt, and freshly ground pepper. Stir again and serve.

9) Quinoa with roasted carrots

Ingredients:
- 250 g of quinoa
- 4-5 carrots
- 4 shallots
- 1/2 tablespoon of cumin
- 1/2 tablespoon of turmeric
- 1 handful of toasted pine nuts
- 1 handful of parsley and very finely chopped celery
- extra virgin olive oil
- salt and pepper

Peel the shallots and halve them; cut the carrots in four lengthwise and then into chunks. Put the vegetables in a pan seasoned with oil, cumin, and salt. Bake at 180 degrees for about 30 minutes, turning them now and then until they are well roasted. Meanwhile, wash the quinoa well in cold water, drain it in a tightly meshed colander and rinse again; drain well and dry briefly in a pan with two tablespoons of oil, turmeric, and pepper.

Pour in boiling water equal to double the quinoa's volume, add salt, cover, and cook over very low heat for 15-20 minutes until the liquid is completely absorbed. Shell the quinoa well and mix it with the vegetables, also collecting their cooking juices, with the pine nuts, celery, and parsley. Serve immediately.

10) Spinach in a pan with dried fruit

Ingredients:
- **500 g of spinach**
- **50 g of dried apples**
- **50 g of raisins**
- **a little pine nuts**
- **1 clove of garlic**
- **extra virgin olive oil as needed**
- **Salt to taste**

Soak the apples and raisins for about 20 minutes in warm water. Clean and wash the spinach. Blanch them in lightly salted water for a few minutes. Drain them by squeezing them well, and cut them coarsely. Fry the garlic in a pan greased with oil, add the spinach, and after a while, the raisins and well-squeezed apples, pine nuts, and salt. Let it cook over high heat for a few minutes, season with salt, and serve the spinach hot.

11) Rice and zucchini croquettes with saffron sauce

Ingredients:

For the croquettes:

- 350 g of rice
- 850 ml of water
- 800 g of zucchini
- 2 tablespoons of oil
- 1 teaspoon of salt
- 1 bunch of parsley
- 1 clove of garlic
- salt and pepper

For the saffron sauce:

- 250 ml of soy milk
- 30 ml of oil
- 30 g of rice flour
- 1 sachet of saffron

Brown the chopped garlic and parsley in a little oil. Add and stew the sliced zucchini with salt and pepper for 10 minutes. Puree about 1/3 of the zucchini. Wash the rice, drain it and cook it in salted water, covered and without stirring, for about 35 minutes. Season the rice with the salt, the zucchini not pureed, stir, and continue cooking for another 5 minutes. Let it cool, then form some meatballs that you will bake in the oven at 200 ° for about 15-20 minutes. To prepare the sauce, brown the flour in a saucepan with the oil, then add the milk. Bring to a boil and let it thicken over low heat, stirring with a whisk. Salt and add the saffron and the zucchini puree.

12) Sweet and sour peppers

Ingredients:
- 2 yellow peppers
- 2 red peppers
- 80 g of raisins
- 100 ml of apple cider vinegar
- 5 tablespoons of oil
- 4 cardamom capsules
- 1-2 tablespoons of chopped parsley
- 1 teaspoon of turmeric
- 1 pinch of Himalayan salt

In a pan with a diameter of 24 cm, heat 200 ml of water with the washed but not soaked raisins, apple cider vinegar, and 2 tablespoons of oil. Meanwhile, clean the peppers well, removing the seeds and white filaments, wash them, and cut them into eight wedges.

Dip them into the boiling liquid along with the cardamom. Cook them for 10 minutes, turn off the stove, season with salt, turmeric, and the remaining oil. Stir and serve sprinkled with chopped parsley.

13) Buckwheat medallions in tomato sauce

Ingredients:
- 200 g of buckwheat
- 1 clove of squeezed garlic
- salt
- ½ tablespoon of curry
- ½ tablespoon of marjoram
- ½ tablespoon of cumin
- breadcrumbs
- extra virgin olive oil for frying

For the sauce
- 1 small onion
- 400 g of tomato puree
- 1 bunch of basil
- salt and pepper
- 10 pitted olives
- 2 tablespoons of oil

Put the buckwheat in a pot with 500 ml of water, a pinch of salt, and bring to a boil. Cover and cook for 10 minutes, then turn off and let cool with the lid on. Add the spices, garlic, and a part of the breadcrumbs; form flattened meatballs, bread them and fry them in boiling oil. Chop and sauté the onion with a little water and oil for about 8-10 minutes; then add the puree, olives, chopped basil, salt, and pepper. Continue cooking for about 30 minutes. Serve the pancakes hot with the sauce.

14) Rice balls with broccoli and almond pesto

Ingredients:

For the stuffing

- already cooked rice
- extra virgin olive oil or seeds for frying

For the batter

- chickpea flour
- water q.s.
- a pinch of salt
- breadcrumbs

For the broccoli and almond pesto

- half a fresh broccoli
- 80 g of almonds
- the juice of half a lemon
- a clove of garlic
- a large tuft of fresh parsley
- Salt to taste.
- extra virgin olive oil as needed

Let's start by preparing the broccoli and almond pesto. Cut your broccoli into small pieces and steam it or cook it in a pot in hot water for a maximum of 10 minutes. Put it in the blender and add the remaining ingredients: the garlic clove into small pieces, the parsley, the lemon juice, the almonds, the salt, and the olive oil. Blend vigorously, help yourself using a little water if necessary (the one used for cooking broccoli, for example), taste, and season with salt. Put the pesto in a large bowl and let the ingredients rest. At this point, we proceed with the preparation and cooking of the meatballs. In a bowl, mix the chickpea flour with water, avoiding the formation of lumps. Mix vigorously until you get a thick and homogeneous batter. Add a pinch of salt. Prepare a dish with the center's breadcrumbs: you can make your breading even tastier by adding chopped aromatic herbs, garlic or onion, sesame seeds, or chopped hazelnuts. Take some rice and form a ball with wet hands that you will dip first in the batter and then pass it in the breadcrumbs. Repeat the operation until the dough is used up.

Prepare a pot with a high bottom and put the oil to heat. Once the temperature is reached, start frying your meatballs for a few minutes until they are golden and place them in a dish lined with absorbent paper. Take a serving dish, place your hot and crunchy meatballs in the center, bring to the table and serve them accompanied by the broccoli and almond pesto sauce.

15) Fennel in orange cream

Ingredients:
- 2 medium fennel
- 1 cup of cashews
- 125 ml of orange juice
- 2 teaspoons of dried mint
- 1 pinch of chilli
- 1 tablespoon of oil
- ½ teaspoon of salt
- 1 teaspoon of agave syrup

Wash the fennel, cut them into four parts, and, using a mandolin, slice them finely. Sprinkle it with salt and let it rest. Meanwhile, prepare the cream. Put the cashews in the blender with the orange juice, mint, chili pepper, oil, salt, and agave syrup and mix until the mixture is fluid and without lumps. Drain the fennel water and season with the cream.

Chapter 6: Soups and salads

1) Oat milk mushroom cream

Ingredients:
- 2 shallots
- 2 tablespoons of flour
- 400 ml of vegetable broth
- 200 ml of oat milk
- 400 g of mushrooms
- 20 g of dried porcini mushrooms
- ½ teaspoon of marjoram
- 1 tablespoon of chopped parsley
- 2 tablespoons of oil
- 100 g of oat flakes
- salt

Rinse the dried mushrooms and soak them in hot water for 30 minutes. Filter the liquid and squeeze the porcini mushrooms, then cut them up. Spread the flakes in a single layer on a baking sheet lined with baking paper, bake them at 180 ° and toast them for 10 minutes, turning them now and then. Let them cool. Meanwhile, you have cleaned the mushrooms with a damp cloth and sliced them. Chop the shallots and put them in a pan with a little broth, marjoram, and a pinch of salt. Let them soften over medium heat, then add the fresh and dried mushrooms. Stir, sprinkle with flour and pour in the hot oat milk without stopping stirring from avoiding lumps. Sprinkle with the rest of the hot broth and the soaking water of the porcini mushrooms.

Cook the soup for about 20 minutes, then blend it by immersion. Season it with salt, season it with oil and transfer it to the soup plates, where you have distributed the toasted flakes. Garnish with parsley and serve.

2) Spelled and potato soup

Ingredients:
- 250 g of spelled
- 3 potatoes
- 1 red onion
- 1 heart of celery
- 2 carrots
- 100 g of peeled tomatoes
- extra virgin olive oil
- salt and pepper

Soak the spelled in cold water overnight. The next day, rinse it and cook it in a pot with one and a half liters of salted water for about 20 minutes. Peel the potatoes and onion, peel the carrot and celery. Cut all the vegetables into cubes or small pieces. In an earthenware pot, first brown a fried onion, celery, and carrots with a salt pinch. Just wilted, add the potatoes and the broth until everything is covered . Stew on low heat. Halfway through cooking, pour in about a liter of broth and continue cooking for 20 minutes. Once cooked, pass the vegetables through a vegetable mill and add the boiled spelled. Mix the ingredients and season with salt and pepper. Serve the soup dressed with raw extra virgin olive oil.

3) Carrot soup with almonds

Ingredients:
- 2 potatoes
- 1 kg of carrots
- 500 g of fennel
- 1 stalk of celery
- 150 g of almonds
- 1 bunch of parsley
- 2-3 tablespoons of sunflower oil

Wash the fennel and celery, potatoes, and carrots; cut the prepared vegetables into small pieces and chop the almonds. Collect everything in a pot. Pour enough water to cover the vegetables by about two fingers. Bring to a boil, reduce the heat; cook for about 30 minutes, remove from heat, and work the mixture with the hand blender until creamy. Season with salt and complete with the washed and chopped parsley and sunflower oil.

4) Pumpkin and cauliflower soup

Ingredients:
- a small pumpkin
- half a teaspoon of salt
- a cup of cauliflower
- a teaspoon of white miso

In a saucepan, arrange diced pumpkin. Cover with water, add salt and cook until the vegetables are well softened. Blend until you get a soft pumpkin cream. In a saucepan of boiling water, cook the pieces of cauliflower for 2-3 minutes. Drain and add them to the pumpkin cream. Dress with white miso. Garnish with parsley and serve.

5) Cream of purple potatoes

Ingredients:
- 600 g of purple potatoes
- 200 g of cooked pumpkin
- 1 dl of oat cream
- 1 stick of celery
- 1 onion
- 1 carrot
- 200 g baguette
- extra virgin olive oil
- 2 cloves of garlic
- salt

Put the onion in a liter of water and boil for the vegetable broth. We combine the cleaned carrot and celery stalk and let it boil for 40 minutes, then filter and prepare the cream. In a saucepan, put the chopped onion with a little oil; when it is golden, add the purple potatoes, washed, peeled, and diced. After about ten minutes, gradually add the broth, stir and cook over moderate heat for about half an hour. Meanwhile, brown the chopped garlic in a pan with plenty of oil, then remove it and brown the bread cut into cubes of about one centimeter.

Pour the cream into the pan with the potatoes, blend everything by immersion, season with salt, and season with oil. We also purée the cooked pumpkin, salt lightly, and let a few small spoonfuls slide over the cream, trying to keep the orange patches spaced apart. Finally, we serve a small bowl accompanied with the croutons to soak.

6) Tasty coleslaw

Ingredients:
- ¼ of white cabbage
- ¼ of red cabbage
- 2 carrots
- 1 teaspoon of brown sugar
- 1 tablespoon of apple cider vinegar
- 5 tablespoons of vegan low-fat mayonnaise
- 1 teaspoon of Dijon mustard
- 1 piece of onion

Wash the two types of cabbage, dry them, and cut them very thin. Rinse the carrots and, with the help of a potato peeler, cut them into slices lengthwise. Mix the vegetables, add the salt, sugar, and vinegar. Stir well and transfer to a colander. Let it macerate for an hour. After this time, squeeze the vegetables and place them in a salad bowl. Stir in the chopped onion and mayonnaise mixed with the mustard. Mix well and serve.

7) Spelled and bean soup

Ingredients:
- 120 g of beans
- 150 g of pearl spelled
- 1-2 tablespoons of extra virgin olive oil
- 1 small leek
- 2 celery sticks
- 1 carrot
- 1 piece of pumpkin
- 1 potato
- about 2 liters of vegetable broth
- 1 bunch of herbs (sage, rosemary, bay leaf)
- 1 pinch of red pepper
- a small sprig of chopped parsley
- 1 teaspoon of salt

Soak the beans for 12 hours; remove the soaking water, cover abundantly with fresh water, bring to a boil; then cook for an hour and a half over low heat, adding salt towards the end of cooking. Take half of the beans with the cooking water and pass them through a vegetable mill. Cut the vegetables into cubes, toss the leek in the oil first for 1-2 minutes and then all the others with the salt and chilli. Add the spelled, the bunch of herbs and the vegetable broth; cook in a covered pot over low heat for 30 minutes. Add the beans (pureed and whole), and continue cooking for another 15 minutes. Let the soup rest for about an hour before serving (but it is also good right away!), Garnish each portion with a drizzle of oil and chopped parsley.

8) Cream of barley

Ingredients:
- 300 g of barley
- 2 l of vegetable broth
- 1 sprig of rosemary
- 1 clove of garlic
- 2 carrots
- 2 sticks of celery with the leaves
- 1 onion
- 1 kohlrabi with leaves
- 6 sprigs of parsley
- 4 tablespoons of soy cream
- 2 teaspoons of turmeric

Soak the barley overnight, then drain and rinse it. Boil the broth with garlic and rosemary without the sprig. Add the barley, lower the heat and cook for 30 minutes. Meanwhile, clean the carrots, celery, and kohlrabi. Cut them into small pieces and add them to the barley. Season with turmeric and pepper. Continue cooking for about 20 minutes. Finally, pass everything to the mixer. Add the soy cream and heat the cream over low heat. Season with salt and serve.

9) Colorful buckwheat salad

Ingredients:
- **300 g of buckwheat**
- **2 bay leaves**
- **250 g of boiled green beans**
- **4 ripe tomatoes**
- **1 large bunch of fresh basil**
- **100 g of green olives**
- **1 small clove of garlic**
- **200 g of canned corn**
- **oil**
- **salt and pepper**

Toast the buckwheat without adding fat and cook it with double the water for 20 minutes: when it boils, lower the heat and cook covered with salt and bay leaf. Drain it and let it cool. Meanwhile, wash the green beans, remove the seeds from the first and chop with the second. Rinse the basil well and blend it with the pitted olives, the chopped garlic in quarters, pepper, salt, and oil. Spread the dressing over the cereal, mix the other ingredients and serve this salad cold.

10) Coconut vegetable stew

Ingredients:

- 1 tablespoon of oil
- 2 cloves of garlic
- 1 fresh red pepper
- 200 g of green beans
- 250 g of cooked black beans
- 2 potatoes
- 400 ml of coconut milk
- the juice of 1 lime
- 1 handful of fresh coriander
- 2 handfuls of roasted cashews, lightly salted
- salt
- water
- cooked rice (optional)

Heat the oil over high heat in a thick-bottomed saucepan. Brown the peeled the cleaned and chopped garlic, red pepper, and potatoes, add salt and leave to flavor briefly, stirring constantly. Lower the heat, stir in the sprouted and chopped green beans, and if necessary, pour a little water, cover, and continue cooking for 5-10 minutes. When the potatoes are tender enough, add the black beans and coconut milk and cook. Once you have reached the consistency of a soft stew, remove from heat, sprinkle with lime juice, season with salt, mix and divide into plates. Complete with cashews and coriander washed and fragmented; serve with rice.

11) Fresh barley salad

Ingredients:
- 300 g of barley
- 800 ml of vegetable broth
- 1 cucumber
- 3 medium ripe tomatoes
- 2 sweet green chillies
- 10 champignon mushrooms
- 1 shallot
- 1 small bunch of basil
- 1 clove of garlic
- 2 tablespoons of sunflower seeds
- the juice of 1 lemon
- 4 tablespoons of oil, salt

Soak the barley overnight. Rinse it and transfer it to a saucepan with the cold broth. Cover and boil it, lower the heat and cook for 40-50 minutes until the liquid runs out. Season the barley with a tablespoon of oil and let it cool. Clean the peppers, cucumber, and tomatoes. Cut the first into rings, the second into cubes, and the third into slices. Put them in a salad bowl. Add the salt and lemon juice. Clean and slice the mushrooms. Add them to the salad along with the finely chopped shallots. Wash the basil, dry it and transfer it to the mixer with the rest of the oil, garlic, and sunflower seeds. Work until you get a homogeneous mixture, helping yourself if needed with a little water. Mix everything with the barley, turn well and let it rest in the fridge for an hour. Serve at room temperature.

12) Peach, parmesan and rocket salad

Ingredients:
- 2 yellow peaches
- 80 g of rocket
- 80 g parmesan
- 7-8 tablespoons of extra virgin olive oil
- 3 teaspoons of black sesame seeds
- salt

Divide the peaches in half, remove the stone and peel them (if they are too ripe, peel them before halving and peeling them); then slice them thinly. Arrange the washed and dried rocket on four plates; distribute the prepared fruits and season the salad with oil and a light sprinkling of salt. Ultimate by distributing in each portion the pecorino reduced to flakes and sesame seeds.

13) Cold avocado soup

Ingredients:
- 1 handful of fresh coriander
- 1 clove of garlic
- a few tufts of chives
- the juice of 1 lime
- a few pinches of cumin powder
- a few pinches of nutmeg
- salt
- black pepper

Combine the peeled and pitted avocados, the peeled and chopped garlic, the cleaned and chopped chives, the lime, the cumin, the nutmeg, salt, and pepper in a blender. Blend, adding cold water in small quantities until you reach a soft consistency. Add the washed and chopped coriander, work the mixture again to mix it, and transfer it to a bowl. Put it in the refrigerator to cool. Serve it in individual bowls, completing, if you like, with a little cream and a few leaves of fresh coriander or chopped chives.

14) Cream of spinach with pine nuts

Ingredients:
- 1 kg of spinach
- 2 shallots
- 500 ml of vegetable broth
- 100 ml of soy milk
- 100 g of creamy tofu
- 2 tablespoons of flour
- 2 tablespoons of pine nuts
- 2 teaspoons of turmeric
- 2 tablespoons of oil
- salt and pepper

Clean the spinach, wash and drain them. Finely chop the shallots and let them soften in a saucepan with a little broth for about ten minutes. Add the flour, stir to avoid lumps, and add the spinach. Add salt, stir briefly and pour in the warmed milk and remaining broth, tofu, and turmeric. Cook for about ten minutes and blend by immersion. Peppered, seasoned with oil, and served garnished with lightly toasted pine nuts and, if desired, with oat cakes.

Chapter 7: Single course

1) Lentil and rice pie

Ingredients:
- 200 g of lentils
- 250 g of rice
- vegetable broth
- 2 shallots
- 2 carrots
- 1 medium potato
- 500 g of celeriac
- 1 bay leaf
- 3 tablespoons of oil
- 2 tablespoons of tamari
- bread crumbs
- 3 tablespoons of sesame
- 1 teaspoon of paprika
- 1 teaspoon of oregano
- salt and chilli

Soak the lentils for a few hours, drain and boil them for about 40 minutes in water with the bay leaf. Salt towards the end. Gather the rice and 600 ml of broth in a saucepan. With the lid on, boil and reduce the heat. Cook until the liquid runs out. Finely chop the shallots and place them in a pan with oregano, chili, and paprika. Salt and add enough water to cover flush. Cook over medium heat, stirring occasionally. After a few minutes, add the potato, carrots, and celeriac cut into cubes. Stir and pour in a little hot broth.

Stew over low heat, adding more hot broth when needed. In the end, transfer the vegetables to the mixer to obtain a thick and creamy mixture, helping you in the case with a little broth. Grease a mold with a bit of oil where you transfer the rice mixed with the lentils. Drizzle with the remaining oil and soy sauce. Cover with vegetable cream and sprinkle with breadcrumbs mixed with sesame. Bake at 180 degrees for about 20 minutes. Serve the pie hot.

2) Ricotta and walnut pie

Ingredients:
- 500 g of ricotta
- 4-5 tablespoons of lightly toasted walnuts
- 2 tablespoons of milk
- 4 nice pinches of saffron stigmas
- 3 tablespoons of marjoram leaves
- salt
- oil for the molds

Infuse the saffron in hot milk for about an hour. Pour the infusion over the ricotta you have sifted into a bowl, add the coarsely chopped walnuts and marjoram, season with salt. Mix all the ingredients to form a cream that you will distribute in the individual round casseroles about 10-12 centimeters wide, greased with a drizzle of oil. Bake for 20 minutes at 180 degrees. When the patties are ready, take them out of the oven and gently remove them from the molds; arrange them in the center of the plates, accompanying them with salads arranged in a crown and possibly dressed with a light vinaigrette.

3) White bean paté with caper pesto

Ingredients:
- 300 g cannellini beans (cooked weight)
- 30 g of onion
- 30 g of Evo oil
- 20 g of salted capers
- 15 g of lemon juice
- 10 g of lemon zest
- a bay leaf

Boil the beans, which you have previously soaked for at least 12 hours, with a bay leaf. Soak the capers in plenty of warm water and leave them to desalt for the entire preparation time. Then reduce them to a puree, mashing them with a fork or blending them with a hand blender. Help yourself with half the oil and lemon juice to make the pate more homogeneous and fluffy. Separately, chop the onion and cut the lemon zest into thin strips. Drain the capers and chop them coarsely. Place the pate on a plate, season it with the remaining extra virgin olive oil, onion, lemon peel, and capers. Serve at the table cold or room temperature, accompanied by slices of toasted bread.

4) Chickpea stew

Ingredients:
- a cup of chickpeas left to soak overnight
- 2 teaspoons of extra virgin olive oil
- 2 carrots
- 2 cloves of garlic
- 2 celery sticks
- 2 bay leaves
- 2-3 tablespoons of miso

Drain the chickpeas and cook them in a pot full of water for about an hour over medium heat. Cut the vegetables and brown them in a pan with oil for about 5 minutes over high heat. Add the vegetables and bay leaves to the beans and simmer until the vegetables are well cooked. Add the miso and cook for a few more minutes. Serve with a sprinkling of chopped parsley.

5) Pasta and cauliflower

Ingredients:
- **350 g of wholemeal short pasta**
- **1 cauliflower of 800 g**
- **400 g of peeled tomatoes**
- **3 tablespoons of oil**
- **2 cloves of garlic**
- **1 teaspoon of marjoram**
- **1 teaspoon of spicy paprika**
- **50 g of Parmesan cheese**

Clean the cauliflower, wash it, divide it into florets and steam it for 10-15 minutes. Meanwhile, put the crushed tomatoes with a fork, chopped garlic, marjoram, paprika, salt in a saucepan. Cook them for about 15 minutes. Add the cauliflower. Cook for a few minutes, stirring. Bring water to boil in a saucepan. When it comes to the boil, cook the pasta for the time indicated on the package. Drain and pour the cauliflower pasta. Grate the cheese, turn the heat back on under the pasta and stir for 1 minute over medium heat. Season with oil, season with salt, and serve.

6) Eggplant stuffed with mushrooms

Ingredients:
- **4 medium eggplants**
- **300 g of champignon mushrooms**
- **1 clove of garlic**
- **1 small bunch of fresh thyme**
- **bread crumbs**
- **3 tablespoons of oil, salt**

Wash and clean the eggplants, dry them and divide them in half lengthwise. Dig them inside with a sharp knife, being careful not to break the shell. Cut the pulp into cubes and cook in a pan with a little water. Add salt, stir for a few minutes over medium heat. Cook for 10 minutes. Clean and slice the mushrooms. Stew them in a pan with the peeled and halved garlic and 1 tablespoon of oil. After 15 minutes on low heat, turn off and add salt. Mix the mushrooms with the eggplant pulp and season with the remaining oil. Season with salt and complete with chopped thyme. Fill the eggplants with this mixture and sprinkle them with breadcrumbs. Arrange them on a baking sheet lined with parchment paper and bake at 190 ° for 40-50 minutes. Serve warm or hot.

7) Rice salad in tomatoes

Ingredients:
- **4 large ripe but firm tomatoes**
- **200 g of brown rice**
- **500 ml of broth**
- **1 spring onion**
- **80 g of mayonnaise)**
- **10 pitted green olives**
- **a few sprigs of fresh marjoram**
- **salt**

Pour the rice and broth into a saucepan. Put the lid on; when it boils, lower the heat and cook for 40-45 minutes. In the last 10 minutes add the green part of the onion, washed and shredded. When cooked, add salt to the rice and let it cool. Wash the tomatoes, remove the top cap, empty them internally and add salt. Mix the mayonnaise with the rice; if the mixture is too dry, add a little tomato pulp (saving the rest for a salad or a sauce). Incorporate a mixture made with the white onion and marjoram. Complete with the chopped olives and stuff the tomatoes with the mixture obtained. Cover them with the cap and let them rest in the fridge for half an hour before serving.

8) Pasta with cherry tomatoes and capers

Ingredients:
- 280 g of wholemeal pasta of your choice
- 12-15 cherry tomatoes, cleaned and quartered
- 4-5 tablespoons of extra virgin olive oil
- half a white onion, peeled and chopped
- 2 spicy green peppers, cleaned and chopped
- 1 generous handful of salted capers
- 1 handful of fresh, clean oregano

Soak the capers in cold water for about 20 minutes, rinse and drain. Cook the pasta in abundant salted water. Meanwhile, heat the oil in a large pan and lightly soften the onion. Add the chilies, tomatoes and cook the capers for 4-5 minutes beforehand. Once the pasta is cooked, drain and add it to the sauce. Stir a couple of minutes, remove from heat, stir and serve.

9) Zucchini stuffed with chickpeas

Ingredients:
- 4 medium-large zucchini
- vegetable broth q.s.
- 250 g of boiled chickpeas
- 2 shallots
- 1 teaspoon of coriander seeds
- 20 g of dried mushrooms
- 1 teaspoon of marjoram
- the juice of 1/2 lemon
- 3 tablespoons of oil
- Salt to taste

Soak the mushrooms in warm water for 30 minutes. Wash the zucchini and steam them whole for 5 minutes. Let them cool, tick them, and cut them in half lengthwise; gently dig them to remove most of the pulp, taking care not to break the peel. Set them aside. Finely chop the shallots and let them soften for a few minutes in a pan, lightly covered with broth. Add the marjoram and the squeezed and thinly sliced mushrooms. Follow with the crushed coriander and salt. Cook for 10 minutes on low heat, finally adds the chickpeas, a tablespoon of oil, and lemon juice. Stir and turn off the heat. Blend by immersion, helping you if needed with a little broth but trying to keep the mixture firm. Transfer it to the zucchini shells, which you will then line up on a baking sheet lined with baking paper. Bake at 180 degrees for about 30 minutes. Serve the dish hot or warm, seasoned with the remaining oil.

10) Rice and peas

Ingredients:
- **200 g of rice**
- **1 Kg of peas**
- **garlic**
- **parsley**
- **extra virgin olive oil**
- **salt and pepper**

Bring salted water to a boil for cooking the rice. Meanwhile, in a pan, cook the shelled peas cold with finely chopped garlic and parsley and a glass of water. When almost cooked, evaporate any excess water, add salt, and season with extra virgin olive oil. Serve the boiled rice with the peas.

11) Pasta with chickpeas and celery pesto

Ingredients:
- **250 g of pasta**
- **150 g of cooked chickpeas**
- **70 g of tender ribs and celery leaves**
- **50 g of linseed or sesame seeds**
- **50 ml of water from pasta or legumes**
- **oil and salt**

Prepare the pesto. Lightly toast the flax (or sesame) seeds in a non-stick pan. After a couple of minutes, turn off the heat. Peel the celery and wash it, dry it and chop it. Put it in the hand blender's jar with the seeds and water from the pasta (or chickpeas). Add lightly salt and stir, gradually adding the oil needed to obtain a soft cream, similar to cream. In the meantime, you will have boiled the pasta al dente. Drain it, mix it with the chickpeas and season with the celery pesto, then serve it.

12) Spaghetti with walnut and basil sauce

Ingredients:
- 400 g of spaghetti
- 100 g of shelled walnuts
- 80 g of pine nuts
- 1 clove of garlic
- 30 g of basil leaves
- 2 tablespoons of grated parmesan
- 3 tablespoons of oil
- salt

Prepare the sauce. Spread the walnuts and half of the pine nuts on a baking tray in a single layer. Bake them at 150 ° for about ten minutes until they are lightly toasted. During this time, stir them a couple of times. Let them cool down and remove the skin by rubbing them. Put them in a mixer with a little salt and chop finely. Add the peeled and chopped garlic, then washed and dried basil, a few tablespoons of hot water. Continue to work the ingredients until they are homogeneous, adding a little more hot water. Complete with oil. Cook the spaghetti in boiling salted water, and season immediately with the walnut and basil sauce. Sprinkle them with the grated Parmesan and serve.

13) Spelled and pistachio flans with carrot and tofu cream

Ingredients:
For the flans:

- 350 g of spelled
- 850 ml of water
- 250 g of shelled pistachios
- 5 tablespoons of extra virgin olive oil
- a bunch of basil
- 1 clove of garlic
- 150 ml of soy cream
- salt and pepper

For the carrot and tofu cream:
- 250 g of fresh tofu
- 250 g of carrots
- 150 ml of soy milk
- 3 tablespoons of sunflower oil
- 2 teaspoons of lemon juice
- 1 teaspoon of paprika and salt

For the pesto, remove the skin from the pistachios by immersing them for a couple of minutes in boiling water. Grind them in the mixer for 1 minute with the oil, the washed and dried basil, and the peeled garlic. Add the cream, salt, pepper, and operate for another minute. Wash the spelled, drain it, and put it in a saucepan with salted water. Bring to a boil and reduce the heat to low.

Cover and continue cooking without stirring for 35-40 minutes. Finally, add the pistachio pesto. Meanwhile, prepare the carrot and tofu cream. Boil the tofu for about 10 minutes in lightly salted water with the peeled and chopped carrots. Drain them and put them in a mixer with the sunflower oil, salt, lemon juice, and paprika; operate and add the soy milk a little at a time until it forms a soft and smooth cream. Oil the molds and fill them with spelled pressing them well with a spoon, let them rest for a few minutes. Bake the flans in the oven at 180 degrees for 40 minutes. Turn the flans over onto serving plates, cover with a couple of tablespoons of cream and serve.

14) Artichoke and lentil cake pan

Ingredients:
- 12 artichokes
- 1 lemon
- 300 g of lentils
- 2 shallots
- 1 sprig of rosemary
- 1 sprig of sage
- 1 teaspoon of thyme
- vegetable broth
- bread crumbs
- 4 tablespoons of oil
- salt

Soak the lentils overnight, rinse them and place them in a saucepan with the chopped rosemary and sage. Cover them with cold water and cook for about 40 minutes. Add salt only at the end. Clean the artichokes, halve them and wash them in water acidulated with lemon juice. Cook them al dente in a pan with the thyme, a tablespoon of oil, and a little water, salt. Be careful not to break them and keep them crunchy. Blend the lentils until the mixture is not too moist. Finely chop the shallots, let them dry in a pan with a tablespoon of oil and a little water. Add the past and let it flavor for a few minutes. Add another tablespoon of oil and stir.

Grease a round mold with high sides, and sprinkle it with breadcrumbs. Form the first layer with half of the artichokes. Pour half of the remaining oil, distribute the legume purée and arrange the rest of the artichokes on the surface. Season with the remaining oil and bake at 190 ° for 10 minutes. Serve the dish hot.

15) Brown rice with ginger

Ingredients:
- **400 g of cooked brown rice**
- **2 spring onions**
- **1 carrot**
- **cabbage 350 g**
- **2 tablespoons of oil**
- **salt**
- **1 piece of ginger root**

Cut the spring onions into rings, the carrot into not too thin matches, and the cabbage into strips. Grease a pan with oil and toss the spring onions with a pinch of salt for a minute. Then add the carrot, cabbage, and another pinch of salt and sauté for another 8-9 minutes, often stirring, until the vegetables begin to be tender (possibly add a couple of tablespoons of water). Then add the cooked rice and a little water to the pan's bottom, cook covered for 5 minutes. Finally, season with the ginger juice, mix, and serve.

Chapter 8: Fish
1) Crispy salmon

Ingredients:
- Salmon fillet (4 of 250 g each) 1 kg
- Bread 100 g
- 1 sprig parsley
- Dill 1 sprig
- Thyme 4 sprigs
- Rosemary 2 sprigs
- Lemon zest 1
- Extra virgin olive oil 50 g
- White pepper in grains 1 tsp
- Salt up to taste

First, prepare the breading: cut the bread into pieces and put it in a mixer, then add the dill, the peeled thyme, the needles of rosemary and parsley. Pour in the oil too, then add the lemon zest, salt and white pepper. Blend until you get a coarse consistency. Now take care of the salmon fillets: remove the skin with a thin-bladed knife and remove the bones with the help of a kitchen tongs, then transfer the fillets to a drip pan lined with parchment paper and cover them with the breading, making it adhere well with your hands. . After covering the fillets evenly, cook in a preheated convection oven at 190 ° for about 20 minutes. After the cooking time, take out and serve your crispy salmon hot!

2) Baked salmon

Ingredients:
- Salmon steaks (4 pieces) 660 g
- Potatoes 170 g
- Lemon zest 1
- Lemon juice 25 g
- Dry white wine 25 g
- Extra virgin olive oil 50 g
- Parsley to chop 1 tbsp
- Salt up to taste
- Black pepper to taste

To prepare the baked salmon, first remove the fish bones with tweezers and check that there are no bones left by sliding a fingertip on the pulp. Remove the spine with a knife, then roll one end on itself and wrap the other end around the slice to obtain a medallion. Tie the medallion with a kitchen string to ensure that it maintains the shape even during cooking and transfer the medallions on a baking sheet lined with parchment paper. Take a fairly regular shaped potato, wash it and cut it into thin slices with a mandolin, without peeling it: the slices must be no more than 1 mm thick otherwise they will not be cooked enough. Now take care of the emulsion: grate the zest of a lemon in a bowl, then add 25 g of lemon juice, oil, white wine, chopped parsley, salt and pepper and mix well with a fork.

Season the salmon medallions with part of the emulsion, then cover them with the slightly overlapping potato discs and sprinkle the potatoes with the remaining emulsion. When the medallions are ready, bake in a preheated static oven at 180 ° for about 20 minutes, then operate the grill at 240 ° and continue cooking for another 3-4 minutes, until the potatoes are golden. After the cooking time has elapsed, remove the cooking string and immediately serve your delicious baked salmon!

3) Salmon rice

Ingredients:
- Rice 350 g
- Salmon steaks 250 g
- Leeks 1
- Extra virgin olive oil q.s.
- 1 clove garlic
- ½ glass white wine
- Parmesan to be grated 20 g
- Salt up to taste
- Black pepper to taste
- Fish broth 500 ml

FOR THE FLAVORED BUTTER
- Butter 80 g
- Marjoram 1 sprig
- Dill 1 sprig
- Thyme 1 sprig
- Lemon zest ½
- Salt up to taste

Prepare the flavored butter by chopping the herbs and grating the lemon zest, allow the butter to soften at room temperature and when it has reached a creamy consistency add the chopped herbs, lemon zest and salt. Meanwhile, clean the salmon steak and cut it into small pieces. Heat a tablespoon of oil in a pan with a clove of whole garlic and brown the salmon bites for 2/3 minutes, add salt and set the salmon aside, removing the garlic.

Now start preparing the risotto: finely chop the leek and sauté it over low heat with two tablespoons of oil in a pan. Pour in the rice and toast it for a few moments over high heat, stirring with a wooden spoon. Deglaze with the counter wine and continue cooking, stirring occasionally, taking care that the rice does not stick, adding the broth (vegetable or fish) a little at a time. Halfway through cooking add the salmon morsels, season with salt if necessary and when the rice is well cooked, remove it from the heat and stir in the herb-flavored butter and a couple of tablespoons of grated cheese, if you like.

4) Mediterranean-style salmon fillets

Ingredients:
- Salmon 800 g
- Dried oregano 1 sprig
- Extra virgin olive oil 30 g
- Salt up to taste
- 1 clove garlic
- Pitted black olives 70 g
- Pickled capers 5 g

In a large bowl, add the peeled and halved garlic and the chopped dried oregano. Add the oil, salt, and mix. Take the salmon steak, remove the bones with tweezers, remove the skin if present; then cut into 4 fillets of equal thickness. Arrange the salmon fillets on a baking dish, and with a teaspoon, arrange the garlic oil. Season with salt, add the black olives and capers. Bake in a preheated static oven at 180 ° for about 15 minutes (if you want to use the convection oven, bake at 160 ° for about 10 minutes). After this time, take out and serve your still warm Mediterranean salmon fillets!

5) Tuna tartare

Ingredients:
- Tuna in slices 450 g
- Oranges 1
- Extra virgin olive oil 40 g
- Salt up to taste
- Black pepper to taste
- Shortcrust pastry 230 g
- Wild fennel 3 sprigs

Start grating the zest of an orange, then cut it in half and squeeze the juice. In a bowl, pour the extra virgin olive oil, the orange juice and its zest. Finely chop the fennel, keeping a few strands aside for the final decoration, add it to the mixture and emulsify with a whisk. Meanwhile, prepare the shortcrust pastry shells. Adjust the emulsion with a pinch of pepper and salt. Prepare the shortcrust pastry shells that will be used to make tartare single portions: roll out the shortcrust pastry (you can use a roll of already made shortcrust pastry), cut out 10 circles of about 10 cm in diameter and line 10 round molds with a diameter of 8 cm , after having buttered them. Prick the bottom with the tines of a fork and cook in white, covered with dried legumes as weight, in the oven at 180 degrees for 10-15 minutes. When they are golden, take them out of the oven, let them cool and turn them out.

Take the tuna steaks: make sure you have bought especially fish. It is recommended to freeze it for 96 hours at -18 degrees and then defrost it for use in the recipe. Rinse and dry the tuna fillets with absorbent paper. Cut them into small cubes half a centimeter thick and place them in a large bowl. Pour the oil and orange emulsion over them and mix so that the tuna is well flavored. Then fill the cakes with one or two tablespoons of tuna tartare and decorate your tartare with a few sprigs of fennel.

6) Tuna in pistachio crust

Ingredients:
- Tuna 600 g
- Poppy seeds 1 tbsp
- Extra virgin olive oil 3 tbsp
- Breadcrumbs 20 g
- Chopped pistachios 50
- Dried tomatoes in oil 30 g
- Salt up to taste

Get yourself a slice of fresh tuna, place the slice in the freezer for at least an hour so that it is more convenient to cut without breaking the fibers. Remove the tuna from the freezer and cut it lengthwise into slices about 2-3 cm thick. Put the tuna slices in a baking dish and drizzle them with the olive oil. Meanwhile, dry the dried tomatoes with a cloth to remove excess oil and chop finely with a knife. Place the chopped pistachios in a bowl, add the chopped tomatoes, poppy seeds and breadcrumbs. Stir to mix the ingredients well and salt the breading to taste. Take the slices of tuna and pass them in the breadcrumbs, pressing well on all sides.

Place a couple of tablespoons of extra virgin olive oil in a non-stick pan and once the necessary heat is reached, add the breaded tuna slices and cook them for 1 minute per side, turning them only once. Do not continue cooking so that the tuna remains pink inside, the tuna must not turn white otherwise the meat will be harder. Remove the pistachio crusted tuna from the pan and cut into 2 cm thick slices, then place them on a serving dish and serve immediately.

7) Spaghetti with tuna

- **Spaghetti 320 g**
- **Tuna in oil (drained) 150 g**
- **Black olives**
- **1 Zucchini**
- **Extra virgin olive oil to taste**
- **Salt to taste**

Start by putting a pot full of water on the heat, season with salt to boil: it will be used to cook the pasta. Drain the tuna fillet from the preservation oil. In a saucepan, brown a diced courgette over low heat with a little oil. When the courgette has wilted, add the tuna and brown it for a couple of minutes, stirring constantly. Meanwhile, cook the spaghetti, while the pasta is cooking, the sauce will also be ready. Drain the spaghetti directly into the pan with the tuna, season with ground pepper, turn off the heat and flavor with fresh basil leaves. Stir and serve your tuna spaghetti hot!

8) Tuna glazed with soy sauce

Ingredients:
- **Tuna fillet 400 g**
- **Red cabbage 500 g**
- **Soy sauce 50 g**
- **White wine vinegar 100 g**
- **Salt up to 30 g**
- **Extra virgin olive oil 20 g**
- **Basil 4 leaves**
- **Sesame seeds 30 g**

Start with the vegetables: julienne the cabbage and place it in a bowl, sprinkling with white wine vinegar and seasoning with salt. Mix the ingredients well and leave to macerate for at least 1 hour, covering with cling film. After this time, drain and rinse the cabbage thoroughly under plenty of running water. Then cook it in a non-stick pan in which you have heated 15 g of oil. Flavored with well washed and dried basil leaves and cover with a lid, cooking over low heat for about 10 minutes. When cooked, the cabbage should still be crunchy. While the cabbage is cooking, dedicate yourself to the tuna. Take a small bowl and pour the soy sauce. Take care of the tuna: make sure you have a fillet already cut down; we advise you to freeze the fillet for at least 96 hours at -18 degrees and then defrost for preparation. Cut the tuna into slices about 4 cm thick. Then place a small bowl next to the soy sauce in which you will have poured the white sesame seeds.

Take a slice of tuna and wet it on all sides with the soy sauce, then completely cover the long sides of the tuna slice with sesame seeds. Repeat the operation with all the slices of tuna. Now take a non-stick pan and pour in 5 g of oil: heat it up and place the slices of tuna on the long sides. Blanch the tuna slices for about 2 minutes, then flip them to cook them on the other side for another 2 minutes. For even cooking, you can also sear the tuna slices sideways, 1 minute on each side. Place a bed of cabbage on the serving dish and arrange the slices of tuna on top of it, accompanying with the soy sauce. Your tuna glazed with soy sauce is then ready to be brought to the table and enjoyed!

9) Baked sardines

Ingredients:
- 18 sardines for a total of about 250 g
- Breadcrumbs 60 g
- Extra virgin olive oil 60 g
- 1 sprig parsley
- Thyme 1 sprig
- 1 clove garlic
- Grated Parmesan cheese 20 g
- Pine nuts 30 g
- Extra virgin olive oil to grease the pan 15g

Pour the breadcrumbs, grated cheese and the crushed garlic clove into a bowl. Rinse, dry and finely chop the parsley; then also add it to the breading and further flavor with the thyme leaves; pour the 60 g of oil and mix everything until you get a uniform mixture. At this point take a baking dish measuring 19x15 cm and sprinkle it with about 15 g of oil. Arrange the sardines horizontally without overlapping each other, salt (not excessively), pepper and cover with half of the previously prepared mixture. Arrange another layer of sardines, taking care to position them vertically (opposite to before), salt, pepper and cover the entire surface with the remaining part of the breading. Finish by decorating the surface with pine nuts. Then cook the sardines in the oven in grill mode at 200 ° for 8 minutes, until they are golden brown. Once cooked, serve the baked sardines while still hot.

10) Spaghetti with anchovies and breadcrumbs

Ingredients:
- **Spaghetti 320 g**
- **Anchovies in oil 30 g**
- **Extra virgin olive oil 20 g**
- **Breadcrumbs 70 g**
- **3 cloves garlic**

Put a pan with water on the heat and bring to a boil: it will then be used to cook the pasta. Meanwhile, pour 10 g of extra virgin olive oil into a pan, then add the peeled garlic cloves and the anchovy fillets drained from the preservation oil. Peel a ladle of hot water and pour it into the pan, so you can melt the anchovies in the best possible way. This will take about 10 minutes so stir often. Meanwhile, in a separate pan pour 10 g of extra virgin olive oil, then add breadcrumbs to toast it and mix everything until the crumbs are golden; keep aside. At this point, cook the pasta in boiling water; you can add at most very little coarse salt if you prefer, as anchovies are very tasty.

Cook the spaghetti for the time indicated on the package. After the time has elapsed, remove the garlic cloves from the saucepan and drain the pasta by dipping it directly into the pan. Add some of the breadcrumbs and mix. If necessary, add a little more cooking water, then serve your spaghetti with the anchovies and garnish with a final sprinkling of breadcrumbs.

11) Orange mackerel

Ingredients:
- Mackerel (4 whole clean) 1200 g
- Orange peel 1
- Extra virgin olive oil q.s.

FOR MARINATING
- Orange juice
- Extra virgin olive oil 30 g
- Dill 2 sprigs
- 2 cloves garlic
- Black peppercorns 1 tbsp
- Salt up to 1 tbsp

Make diagonal cuts on the sides of the mackerel and set aside. Take care of the ingredients for the marinade: with the back of the spoon, crush the peppercorns so they will release their aroma better, then squeeze the juice from the oranges. Peel and thinly slice the garlic. Grease a baking dish with oil, place the mackerel on top and season them on the surface with another drizzle of oil, the peppercorns, salt, scented with the sprigs of dill and flavored with the slices of garlic. Finally, sprinkle the fish with half of the orange juice, cover with plastic wrap and leave to marinate for 2 hours in the refrigerator.

After the marinating time, go to cooking: heat a pan with a drizzle of olive oil and, when it is hot, lay the fillets. Let them cook over high heat for 4 minutes without touching them, then turn them, sprinkle them with the remaining orange juice and continue cooking for another 2 minutes. Once the sauce has congealed and the mackerel are well flavored, serve them immediately garnishing them with grated orange zest on the surface.

12) Mackerel in foil

Ingredients:
- Mackerel (2 clean mackerel)
- Celery 90 g
- Yellow peppers 70 g
- Eggplant 50 g
- Lemons 1
- Basil to taste
- Extra virgin olive oil q.s.
- Salt up to taste

Chop the celery and cut it into cubes, then cut the eggplants into slices and cut into cubes. Remove the internal seeds and the stalk of the pepper and cut it first into strips and then into cubes. Transfer all the cut vegetables to a bowl, scented with fresh basil leaves and season with oil, salt. Now place each clean mackerel on a 35x31 cm sheet of parchment paper, fill the belly of the mackerel with a spoonful of vegetables and then distribute the rest around the fish. Season the fish with a drizzle of olive oil. Wash the lemon and cut into thin slices, then place 3 lemon slices on top of each mackerel. Now close the parcel by lifting the flaps of parchment paper and placing them on top of the fish, then seal well by folding the sides. Place the packets on a baking tray lined with parchment paper and bake in a preheated static oven at 200 ° for 20 minutes. When cooked, take your mackerel in foil out of the oven and serve hot.

13) Swordfish carpaccio with green and pink pepper

Ingredients:
- Swordfish 500
- Semi-skimmed milk 250 g
- Pink peppercorns 5
- Green peppercorns 10
- Extra virgin olive oil 50 g
- Himalayan salt (pink) 5 g

Start by cutting the swordfish slices. Cut the swordfish steak into 16 slices of about 30 g each and 3-4 mm thick. To facilitate the operation, keep the swordfish steak to compact it in the freezer for an hour before slicing it. If you don't have a slicer available, buy the swordfish already cut into slices for the carpaccio or have it cut in your trusted fish shop. Remove the skin of the swordfish with a knife and arrange the slices in a baking dish. Start preparing the marinade: pour the milk and oil into a bowl. Add the green peppercorns, pink pepper and pink Himalayan salt. Emulsify the mixture with a whisk to mix all the ingredients. Pour the marinade into the pan where you have placed the swordfish slices and cover with plastic wrap.

The carpaccio must marinate in the refrigerator for at least 4 hours. After this time, remove the swordfish carpaccio from the fridge and, with the help of a spatula, lift the slices of swordfish one by one, draining the marinade a little, and place them in an ovenproof dish. Bake at 180 degrees for no more than 5 minutes, so that the the fish releases the absorbed marinade. Stir in the swordfish carpaccio with green and pink pepper before serving.

14) Cod fillet with ginger

Ingredients:
- Cod fillet 400 g
- Salt up to taste
- Black pepper to taste
- Extra virgin olive oil 50 g
- Lime zest 1
- Lime juice 10 g
- Fresh ginger (pulp) 20 g
- Mint a few leaves

FOR THE RICE
- Basmati rice 200 g
- Coconut milk 400 g
- Water 200 g
- Coarse salt 1 tbsp
- Cinnamon sticks 1
- Curry 1 tsp

Grate the lime zest in a bowl and squeeze it into juice and pour 10 g into the same bowl. Peel the ginger and grate it, then collect the pulp with a spoon and place it in the bowl with the lime, pour in the olive oil and stir to mix the sauce. Take the cod fillets and place them on a baking sheet lined with parchment paper, salt them and spread the sauce on the surface. Bake in a preheated static oven at 220 ° for 25 minutes. Meanwhile, prepare the rice: pour the basmati rice into a pan, add the coconut milk, the coarse salt, the curry and a stick of cinnamon.

Pour in the water, cover with the lid and bring to a boil, then lower the heat and cook for 15 minutes until the liquids are completely absorbed. When the rice has absorbed the liquids, turn off the heat and remove the cinnamon stick. Meanwhile, the cod will be cooked, take it out of the oven and serve it accompanied with the spiced basmati rice, garnishing with mint leaves.

Chapter 9: Dessert

1) Buckwheat and dark chocolate cake

Ingredients:
- 100 g dates
- 200 g buckwheat
- 60 g bitter cocoa
- 90 g 95% dark chocolate
- Grated orange peel to taste
- 140 g tofu
- ½ teaspoon of agar agar

Soak the buckwheat for 24 hours, then drain and place in a sprouter. Rinse twice a day for 2-3 days, and as soon as it begins to sprout, place in the dryer basket at 42 ° for 8 hours. Blend the sprouted and dried buckwheat, dates, vanilla, and grated orange zest at maximum power. Add the tofu and continue blending. Separately, dissolve the agar agar in cold water and add to the mixture, mixing again. Add the dark chocolate in pieces and bring to a boil for a few minutes. Pour the mixture into a square shape, a level well, and store in the freezer for 3 hours. When the cake is ready, sprinkle with cocoa. Let it rest out of the freezer for at least half an hour.

2) Apple and pear chutney with ginger and spices

Ingredients:
- 200 g of apples
- 200 g of golden onions
- 150 g of ripe but firm pears
- 40 g of whole cane sugar
- the juice of ½ lemon
- 140 ml of apple cider vinegar
- 4 cm of freshly chopped ginger
- ½ c of dried ginger powder
- ½ c of powdered cumin
- 100 ml of water, salt

Peel and cut the apples and pears into small pieces. Gather them in a thick-bottomed saucepan with the peeled and thinly sliced onions; add the rest of the ingredients and mix. Cook over medium heat for about 40 minutes, stirring often. If necessary, wet with a little water. Continue cooking until you have reached the consistency of a jam. Pour the still warm chutney into the jars and consume it within a week, keeping it in the refrigerator anyway.

3) Rice cream flavored with ginger, turmeric and cinnamon

Ingredients:
- **250 g of gluten free rice biscuits**
- **80 g toasted hazelnuts**
- **500 g rice milk**
- **40 g starch**
- **3 cm cinnamon**
- **8 g of fresh turmeric**
- **20 g fresh ginger**
- **70 g brown sugar**
- **500 g of clean pumpkin**
- **100 g of cane sugar**
- **3 cm cinnamon**
- **water q.s.**

Chop the biscuits and half of the hazelnuts. Heat the rice milk with the cinnamon, which you will then remove. Grate the turmeric and ginger, put them in a kitchen towel, and squeeze them in the milk. When the milk is hot, add the starch and sugar, stirring with a whisk, and cook until the cream has thickened. Let it cool down. Dice the pumpkin and put it in a saucepan with the sugar, cinnamon, and 33 cl of water. Cook until the pumpkin is soft, then blend it with the blender and let it cool. Compose the cake in layers, alternating the biscuits, compote, and cream. As a topping, use the remaining chopped hazelnuts.

4) Beetroot brownies

Ingredients:
- **2 boiled beets**
- **200 g semi-wholemeal flour**
- **100 g dark chocolate (80-90%)**
- **50 g extra virgin olive oil**
- **50 g rice malt**
- **16 g yeast**
- **flaked almonds to taste**
- **1 handful of toasted hazelnuts**

Grate the beets, melt the chocolate in a bain-marie, add the oil, the malt, add the beets and mix everything. Add the sifted flour and baking powder. Mix well until the mixture is quite thick and soft. At this point, add the toasted hazelnuts and coarsely cut them with a knife. Transfer the dough to a previously greased square baking dish (about 30-40 cm). Bake in a preheated oven at 180 ° for about 30 minutes.

5) Greedy glasses

Ingredients:
- **200 g of fresh blueberries**
- **4 heaping tablespoons of sugar-free blueberry jam**
- **2 tablespoons of organic apple juice**
- **500 ml of organic soy yogurt**
- **75 g of oat flakes**
- **75 g of pine nuts**

Clean and wash the blueberries. Blend them with half the yogurt and distribute them in 4 tall glasses. Heat the jam with the apple juice over low heat and divide it into glasses. Cover with the remaining yogurt and let it cool in the fridge for about an hour. Meanwhile, spread the oats and pine nuts on a baking sheet lined with parchment paper and toast them in the oven at 160 ° for about ten minutes, turning them now and then. Let them cool. Sprinkle with the mixture of pine nuts and oats, and serve immediately.

6) Soft blueberry pie

Ingredients:
- **250 g semi-wholemeal flour**
- **200 g of soy drink**
- **Juice and grated zest of 1 lemon**
- **16 g yeast**
- **50 g extra virgin olive oil**
- **50 g rice malt**
- **1 pinch of salt**
- **250 g blueberries**

Gather the flour, yeast, salt, lemon zest in a bowl; mix everything. Combine the soy drink, lemon juice, oil, and malt. Stir well until you get a velvety, lump-free consistency. Now add the blueberries. Transfer the dough to a previously greased loaf pan (about 30 cm). Bake in a preheated oven at 180 ° for about 30-40 minutes. The toothpick test is recommended to verify internal cooking. Let the cake cool before enjoying it. Keep inside a container for three days.

7) Lactose-free strawberry ice cream

Ingredients:
- 500 g of clean organic strawberries
- the juice of 1/2 lemon
- 100 g of rice syrup
- 260 ml of unsweetened rice milk

Cut the strawberries, sprinkle them with the lemon juice and rice syrup, mix and let them rest in the refrigerator for half an hour. After this time, blend the mixture briefly with the rice milk. Leave it to cool for another half hour. Operate the ice cream maker and pour the mixture. It will take between 20 and 25 minutes to get good ice cream, be divided into cups or glasses, and be enjoyed immediately.

8) Pudding with pears and chocolate

Ingredients:
- **500 g vegetable soy drink**
- **3 large pears**
- **3 tablespoons of corn starch**
- **5 g of agar agar**
- **1 pinch of salt**
- **1 teaspoon of vanilla**
- **100 g 99% dark chocolate**
- **Chopped pistachio to taste**

Peel and wash the pears, cut them into slices, and steam them. Put the vegetable drink, agar agar, salt, vanilla, and the starch in a saucepan. Blend everything, add the cooked pears and blend again. Put on the fire, add the chopped chocolate and continue stirring. As soon as it starts to boil, turn off the heat. Put the chopped pistachios on the bottom of a pudding mold. Pour the mixture and let it cool for a few hours at room temperature. Then keep in the refrigerator.

9) Coconut balls

Ingredients:
- **1 cup of cashews**
- **5 dates**
- **grated coconut to taste**
- **rice milk to taste**

Pitted the dates, cut them into small pieces, put them in a robot together with the cashews, and blended them finely. With your hands, form balls, compacting them well. Let them rest for half an hour in the fridge. Meanwhile, mix a little coconut with two tablespoons of rice milk. Take the balls back and roll them in this mixture until they are evenly covered. Finally, put them in the paper cups and serve them.

10) Pear and cinnamon cake

Ingredients:
- 140 g of type 0 wheat flour
- 160 g of millet flour
- 1 p of sea salt
- ½ teaspoon of yeast
- 4 medium pears (2 quite ripe, 2 firmer)
- about 160 ml of rice milk
- 100 ml of oil
- 180 g of rice malt
- ½ teaspoon of ground cinnamon

Begin to heat the oven to 180 ° C. In the meantime, combine the wheat and millet flour in a bowl, the sea salt, yeast and mix well. Clean and peel the pears and cut only the two firmest into thin slices. Set the other two pears aside. Line a pan 20-22 cm in diameter with baking paper and arrange the pear slices on the bottom, overlapping them so that there are no gaps. Then cut the two more ripe pears into small pieces and place them in a mixer bowl. Add the rice milk, the oil, the malt, and the cinnamon and blend well until you obtain a smooth mixture which you will combine with the dry ingredients previously mixed, mixing briefly. Pour everything into the pan on the slices of pear. Bake and cook for 40-45 minutes. Finally, remove the cake from the oven, let it cool for 5-10 minutes before serving it with a vegetable cream sauce sweetened with a few tablespoons of rice malt of about.

11) Vegan apple pie

Ingredients:
- 3 apples
- 250 g of type 1 wheat flour
- 60 g of raisins
- 60 g of almonds
- About 250 ml of apple juice
- 50 g of corn oil
- 1 teaspoon of cinnamon
- grated lemon peel
- 1/2 sachet of baking powder
- 1 pinch of salt

Soak the raisins. In a bowl, put the dry ingredients: flour, chopped almonds, lemon peel, cinnamon, and salt; stir with care. In another, gather the apple juice, the oil, the raisins, the peeled and chopped apples; mix them well, and mix them with the other container's contents. Mix the mixture carefully, roll it out in a pan; bake at 180 degrees for about 50-60 minutes. Check the cooking with a toothpick: if it comes out dry, turn off the oven. Let the cake rest briefly, unmold it, and let it cool completely on a wire rack before enjoying.

12) Plum and fig balls

Ingredients:
- **100 g of pitted dried plums**
- **100 g of dried figs**
- **50 g of chopped hazelnuts**
- **cocoa**

Put the plums, figs, and hazelnuts in the mixer. Knead them until you get a homogeneous mixture from which you will obtain slightly larger balls of hazelnuts with the shell. Roll them well in cocoa and immediately arrange them in paper cups. They are ready to be served!

13) Cookies with apple heart

Ingredients:

For the shortcrust pastry
- an egg
- 100 g of cane sugar
- half a bag of yeast
- semi-wholemeal flour to taste
- a coffee glass of extra virgin olive oil
- grated orange peel

For the apple filling
- 3 apples
- 2 teaspoons of powdered ginger
- the juice of half a lemon
- 2 tablespoons of brown sugar

In a bowl, put the egg, brown sugar, grated orange peel, and olive oil. Mix the ingredients with a fork in a circular and continuous pattern until you get a homogeneous and creamy mixture. Stir in the yeast and mix. At this point, add the sifted flour a little at a time, always mixing it with a fork in the bowl. You will see the dough gradually transform, acquire body and shape while remaining soft. For the recipe's success, this is an important step: consider mixing the flour at the rate of a spoon at a time until your liquid and creamy dough become more compact but not hard. Transfer it to a lightly floured pastry board and knead.

When it no longer sticks to your hands, your pastry will be ready. Give it a ball shape and place it in the refrigerator for 30 minutes. Peel and dice the apples, put them in a bowl, add the lemon juice, the ginger powder, and the sugar. Mix well and pour into a non-stick pan. Cook for about 10 minutes (the time varies depending on the quality of the apples chosen) over moderate heat until you get a fragrant and creamy mixture. Leave to cool. Take the pastry, roll it out finely and form circles you will use to shape your cookies. Everything is ready to assemble the ingredients: you will need a bowl with a little water to seal the edges of the biscuits and prevent the contents from escaping: take a pastry base, put the apple filling in the center, with your index finger wet with water moisten the edges of the two pastry bases; then seal the two edges by pressing on them to push the filling towards the center and prevent it from coming out during cooking. With the help of a fork, decorate the edge with light pressure. Repeat until all ingredients are used up. Put the biscuits in a baking tray covered with parchment paper and bake them for 15 minutes at 180 °. A sprinkle of powdered sugar and they are ready ... soft, healthy, and very tasty.

14) Carrot cake

Ingredients:
- **200 g of wholemeal flour**
- **80 g of almonds**
- **80 g of raisins**
- **200 g of carrots**
- **100 g of rice malt**
- **4 tablespoons of sunflower oil**
- **1 orange**
- **3 tablespoons of corn starch**
- **1 teaspoon of yeast**
- **½ teaspoon of natural vanilla**
- **soya milk**
- **1 pinch of salt**

Wash the orange, grate the zest and squeeze the juice. Put the first in a bowl together with the flour, finely ground almonds, starch, yeast, vanilla, and salt. Stir. Mix the oil, malt, and orange juice in a bowl. Gradually add them to the dry ingredients. Complete with grated carrots and rinsed raisins. If the dough is too firm, dilute it with a little soy milk. Line a square mold of about 20 cm on each side with baking paper. Transfer the mixture, level it, and bake at 180 degrees for about 45 minutes. Check the cooking with a toothpick, which must come out dry. Let the cake cool in the pan, turn it out of the mold, and let it cool.

15) Chocolate cake

Ingredients:
- 80 grams of unsweetened cocoa powder
- 100 grams of coconut flour
- 300 g 0 flour
- 100 gr of hazelnuts
- 150 ml of seed oil
- 350 grams of rice or soy milk
- 150 g of cane sugar
- a sachet of vanilla yeast for cakes

In a blender, finely chop the hazelnuts and place them in a large bowl. Add the unsweetened cocoa, coconut flour and flour, sugar, and vanilla yeast. Mix these ingredients vigorously with your hands, mixing them well together. Then add the vegetable milk and mix the mixture with the help of a spoon. Also, add the seed oil: the result must be a soft, not liquid compound. Line a cake pan with parchment paper and spread the cocoa mixture starting from the center towards the outer sides, and spread all the product well in the pan. You can put some chopped hazelnuts or almonds on top of the cake for decoration. Place in a preheated oven at 180 ° for 40 minutes. Remove from the oven and sprinkle the cake while still hot with a coconut flour cascade or, if you prefer, powdered sugar. Few genuine ingredients that, when mixed, give a great result. Excellent for those intolerant to dairy products and to let everyone discover a lively and tasty vegan diet.

Conclusion

Acid reflux is a stomach related or digestive disorder that creates irritation and a restless condition for a person. The main reason behind this issue is poor digestion, improper food intake, lack of sleep, and inactivity. An increase in obesity and other health complications can cause acid reflux. In this chronic disorder, a person feels heartburn and feels like their food is not properly being digested. Stomach acid and food reverse into the food canal that causes an inability to perform the task and continuous burp can affect a person's productivity as well. As per the consultants, it is necessary to treat the acid reflux at the initial stage with food intake, exercise, and diet control by reducing the weight or following proper medication. It not treated well, then it may cause further health complications like cancer or ulcers as well. To get quick relief from acid reflux, it is necessary to adopt certain dietary changes like taking small meals instead of full meals, following an exercise routine, reducing citrus intake, limiting spicy and fried food intake, and reducing weight.

At the initial stage of acid reflux, it can be treated and prevented with healthy and organic food choices. It also requires a proper medical checkup; this helps to find out how severe the problem is. Consulting doctors and taking their advice for the treatment and precautions is a necessary step a person has to take to avoid gastric acid reflux. In this book, a number of healthy and organic recipes are mentioned that will help a person to enjoy good food and relief in acid reflux conditions as well.

Gastritis Diet Cookbook

Introduction

Gastritis is used to describe a group of disorders with one feature in common, inflammation of the gastric mucosa. Today, in fact, in addition to being a discomfort that affects men and women of every race, age, and social rank, gastritis manifests itself in different guises: some patients suffering from gastritis complain of simple and temporary heartburn; in others, however, the disorder causes aerophagia, dyspepsia, loss of appetite, up to degenerate into severe and disabling symptoms such as diarrhea, abdominal cramps, meteorism, halitosis, and vomiting. The triggering cause heavily conditions the type of symptoms and the intensity with which they occur. Fortunately, in most cases, mild gastritis is quickly remedied by lifestyle correction.

Other times, however, where the disease takes on a chronic or particularly aggressive connotation, the therapy must be more drastic. In both cases, especially if intense, the malaise experienced must not be neglected but submitted to the attention of the doctor, both to avoid suffering unnecessarily and because, albeit in a minority of people, the onset of heartburn, cramps, and abdominal pain can be a sign of a more serious condition that can pose significant risks to overall health. Let's find out the different conditions that can cause it, the most common symptoms useful for recognizing it, the possible treatments to cure it, and a healthy diet.

Chapter 1: What is Gastritis?

Gastritis is an acute or chronic disorder characterized by inflammation of the stomach walls, accompanied by gastric pain, nausea, cramps, and bloating. Often, gastritis is not a consequence of just one factor, being the multifactorial disorder, dependent on multiple causes. Not surprisingly, many times, at the root of the problem, there is a genetic predisposition that is added to an unbalanced diet and an incorrect lifestyle. Stress should also be considered an etiological factor, which today is practically omnipresent in the Western population, affecting both sexes of all ages indiscriminately. A lack of food education, climate change, a sedentary lifestyle, infections, smoking, and the frenetic pace of work can also contribute to potentiate gastritis.

Classification and causes

The stomach walls are generally protected by a mucous membrane that acts as a barrier against the acids responsible for digestion. The acids present are so corrosive that, in the absence of adequate protection, they would end up digesting the stomach itself; if this barrier is weakened, the digestive juices can therefore damage and inflame the stomach walls, causing gastritis. Among the various causes we find:

Helicobacter pylori infection

Infection caused by the bacterium helicobacter pylori is the leading cause of the appearance of gastric ulcers and is also responsible for numerous cases of gastritis, in most cases chronic. It is estimated that half of the world's population has been infected with this bacterium, transmitted from person to person. However, most infected people do not suffer from infection complications, but in some of them, the bacterium can tear the stomach's internal mucosa, thus modifying the gastric walls. It is unknown why only some people suffer from Helicobacter pylori infection (about 20% of the total). Still, doctors believe that vulnerability to the bacterium may be hereditary or is caused by the wrong lifestyle, for example, from smoking and high levels of stress. The H. pylori are contagious, but the exact transmission way has not yet been clarified; the man seems to be the only reservoir in nature for the bacterium. . In support of the hypothesis of oral transmission is the fact that the bacterium has been isolated in plaque and especially in saliva; it is not clear whether the mouth is a random passage (for example caused by regurgitation or vomiting) or not.

Anti-inflammatories and other substances

A chronic and/or excessive use of non-steroidal anti-inflammatories can cause gastritis, both acute and chronic; the abuse of these medicines can reduce the amount of a fundamental substance that helps protect the internal mucosa of the stomach, thus exposing the patient to the development of problems. Stomach problems are less likely if you take them sporadically.

Anti-inflammatories are responsible for about 20% of gastritis cases. Together with anti-inflammatories, other substances are also responsible for some cases, such as:

Alcohol

which can irritate and corrode the gastric mucosa, making the stomach more vulnerable to digestive juices

Bile

The fluid substance that contributes to the digestion of fats, produced by the liver and stored inside the gallbladder; under normal conditions, a valve prevents bile from moving up to the stomach from the intestine, but if this does not function properly, the fluid can flow back into the stomach, causing inflammation and chronic gastritis.

Autoimmune gastritis

In this form of gastritis, the immune system mistakenly attacks healthy stomach cells, mistaking them for a threat to fight. Autoimmune gastritis occurs more frequently in patients suffering from other autoimmune diseases and especially in the elderly population; it is generally not erosive.

Other causes

Stress

Understood as a psychosomatic reaction to situations such as traumatic injuries, serious illnesses, severe burns, and the need to undergo major surgery, which can favor the appearance of nervous gastritis. The exact cause of why this occurs is unknown; it is hypothesized that it may be related to the decreased blood flow to the stomach.

Coffee and spicy foods

To date, there is no scientific evidence that they can cause problems, but it is certainly advisable to avoid them in case of pre-existing symptoms.

Incorrect lifestyle

Bad habits, such as smoking or eating unhealthy foods, are a significant cause of gastritis.

Symptoms

The symptoms of indigestion are the best known and generally resolve positively within a few hours. However, it is a good idea to contact your primary care physician when they last for several days or weeks. If gastritis symptoms arise after taking certain medicines, it is good to report this promptly to your doctor. It is equally important to contact the healthcare professional as soon as possible if you notice traces of blood in the vomit and stools (when the bleeding has gastric origins, the stools are particularly dark).

Common gastritis symptoms

- Bad breath
- Bitter mouth
- Stomach ache
- Weight loss
- Dysphagia
- Dyspepsia
- Hemorrhage (symptom of hemorrhagic gastritis)
- Fever (rare)
- Dark stools
- Flatulence

- Lack of appetite
- Meteorism (swollen belly)
- Nausea
- Feeling of abdominal fullness after eating
- He retched

Chronic gastritis symptoms

- Formation of ulcers
- Halitosis
- Heartburn,
- Anorexia,
- Blood in stool and vomit

Complications

All the variants of gastritis require therapy, which can be simply behavioral, therefore based on incorrect eating habits or life, or pharmacological. In case of lack of treatment, gastritis symptoms can worsen, weighing heavily on the patient's health. Among the most frequent complications associated with gastritis, we remember:

- Gastric ulcers
- Stomach bleeding
- Perforations of the stomach
- Pernicious anemia, possible complication of atrophic gastritis
- Hyperhomocysteinemia due to vitamin B12 deficiency, a possible complication of atrophic gastritis
- Increased risk of gastric cancer, complication from autoimmune atrophic gastritis or untreated H. pylori-dependent gastritis
- Hypovolemic shock and death (extremely rare complications, resulting from untreated hemorrhagic gastritis)

A correlation was also highlighted between autoimmune atrophic gastritis and other serious diseases: Hashimoto's thyroiditis, thyrotoxicosis, myxedema, Addison's disease, and type I diabetes.

Chapter 2: Diagnosis and treatment

Diagnosis

If you think you suffer from gastritis, the first doctor who will visit you will probably be your doctor or a general practitioner; however, in some cases, already when you schedule the visit, you could be directed to a doctor specialized in the treatment of digestive system disorders (gastroenterologist). The doctor will probably arrive at a gastritis diagnosis after asking you about your previous illnesses and thoroughly examining you. Still, you will have to undergo special tests to understand your disorder's cause in some cases. Among the possible exams we mention:

Blood tests: Your doctor will probably prescribe blood tests aimed at discovering the presence of antibodies to H. pylori. If the test is positive, it means that you have come into contact with the bacterium during your life, but this does not necessarily mean that there is an infection in progress. Blood tests can also show anemia, which can be caused by gastric bleeding linked to gastritis.

Breath test: This simple test can help to understand if an H. pylori infection is ongoing.

Stool examination: This examination aims to highlight the presence of H. pylori in a sample of your stool. A positive test indicates an infection in progress. Doctors may also check for blood in the stool, a symptom of gastric bleeding linked to gastritis.

X-ray of the upper gastrointestinal tract: The x-ray of the stomach and small intestine is done to discover the signs of gastritis and other digestive system problems. It is usually performed after taking a liquid (barium) that goes to coat the internal mucous membranes of the digestive system, making them stand out better on the radiographic film (opaque enema).

Gastroscopy: This procedure allows the doctor to check if there are abnormalities in the upper gastrointestinal tract that are not detectable with an X-ray. During the examination, the doctor inserts a thin and flexible tube with a light source at one end (endoscope) through the mouth: the tube is made to descend towards the esophagus, stomach, and the initial section of the small intestine. Before swallowing the endoscope, the throat is usually anesthetized, and particular medications with a calming effect are administered. If a part of the gastrointestinal tissue looks abnormal, the doctor can remove a small sample (biopsy) using the instruments inserted inside the endoscope. The sample is then sent to the laboratory, where a pathologist will analyze it. Endoscopy usually lasts 20 to 30 minutes, but you will not normally be discharged until the drugs' effect ceases (generally after one or two hours). The risks of this surgery are infrequent: we remember gastric bleeding and perforation of the stomach walls. The most frequent complication is a slight sore throat due to having swallowed the endoscope.

Treatment

The cure of gastritis depends on the specific trigger, for example:

-the acute form, caused by drugs or alcohol, can be alleviated by suspending the use of the responsible substances;

-the chronic form caused by H. pylori infection is treated by eradicating the bacterium through antibiotic polytherapy. Most therapeutic programs include drugs that treat stomach acid to decrease the severity of symptoms and encourage the stomach's healing process.

Treatment of stomach acid

Gastric acids irritate the inflamed tissues of the stomach, causing pain and worsening inflammation. Precisely for this reason, most gastritis therapies include drugs that reduce or neutralize stomach acid. Among them, we mention:
- Antacids. Antacids available at pharmacies without a prescription, in liquid or tablet form, are a frequent therapy for mild gastritis cases.

- Antacids neutralize stomach acids and can quickly relieve pain.
- Anti-ulcer drugs (or anti-H2 antihistamines). If antacids are not sufficient, your doctor may advise you to take an anti-ulcer medication, which will reduce the amount of acid produced by the stomach.
- Acid pump inhibitor drugs. The so-called proton pump inhibitors reduce acidity by blocking the tiny pumps' action inside the stomach cells that secrete acidic juices.

Treatment of H. pylori infection

Doctors follow various therapeutic programs to treat H. pylori infection, mostly based on a combination of two antibiotics and a proton pump inhibitor. In some cases, bismuth is also added. Antibiotics destroy the bacterium, while the proton pump inhibitor relieves pain and nausea, treats inflammation, and can increase antibiotics' effectiveness. To ensure that H. pylori have been eliminated, your doctor may test you again at the end of your therapy.

Lifestyle and DIY remedies

Digestive problems can occur for many reasons, including some lifestyle factors that you can control yourself. In general, to keep the digestive system in good condition, doctors recommend:

- Follow a proper diet. How you eat is just as important as the food you eat. Moderate portions, eat at regular times, and try to relax during meals. Avoid irritating foods (spicy, hot, sour, fried, fatty) and alcohol.
- Maintain a healthy weight. Digestive problems can occur regardless of weight. However, heartburn, bloating, and constipation tend to affect overweight people more often. Gaining and maintaining a healthy weight can often help prevent or subside these symptoms.

- Get plenty of exercises. Aerobic activity that improves breathing and heartbeat also stimulates the intestinal muscles' activity, helping you eliminate waste from the intestine faster. We recommend that you do at least 30 minutes of aerobic exercise a day, on most days of the week. Before starting, it is advisable to consult a doctor.
- Keep stress under control. Stress increases the risk of heart attacks and heart attacks, depresses the immune system, and can trigger or aggravate skin problems. As for the digestive system, it increases the production of gastric

acids and slows down digestion. Stress is unavoidable for most people, so the secret is learning how to manage it effectively: the task is easier if you eat a nutritious diet, get enough sleep, exercise regularly, and try healthy ways to relax. If relaxing is a problem, consider taking a meditation, yoga, or tai chi course. These disciplines can help you concentrate, reduce anxiety, and reduce physical tension. Also, therapeutic massage can loosen tight muscles and calm exhausted nerves.

Before taking any treatment, go to your family doctor. The doctor will be able to advise you on the correct therapy to be undertaken.

Prevention

In some cases, H. pylori infection is inevitable, but these tips will help you decrease the chances of being affected by gastritis:

- Limit the use of alcohol or avoid it altogether. Alcohol abuse can irritate and erode the gastric mucosa, causing inflammation and bleeding.
- Don't smoke. Smoking interferes with the protective mucosa's action, making the stomach more prone to gastritis and ulcer. Furthermore, smoking increases stomach acidity, slows down the healing process, and is one of the main risk factors for stomach cancer. Despite everything, quitting smoking is not easy, especially if you have smoked for years. Ask your doctor for advice on methods that can help you stop.
- Change analgesics. If possible, avoid anti-inflammatories. These drugs can cause stomach inflammation or make existing irritation worse.

Chapter 3: Diet

Scrupulous attention to nutrition is undoubtedly the first step for a correct management of the disorder; if episodes of gastritis or stomach acid are frequent, eating lighter and more frequent meals can be of great help because it reduces the effects of gastric hyperacidity. All those foods with irritating power should then be avoided, especially spicy, acidic, fried, or fatty ones, and excessively abundant meals should also be avoided.

What are the most relevant diet tips for gastritis?

The diet for gastritis is based primarily on compliance with some elementary rules; for example, respecting the rules of behavior, changing the composition and size of meals, respecting the list of recommended foods, and limiting/avoiding products not recommended. Here are the most important tips:

- Eat your meals in an environment that promotes relaxation. Chewing, digestion, and gastritis improve as nervous tension decreases.
- Prevent the consumption of meals in conditions of significant nervousness and fatigue
- Eat at regular times, never skipping a meal or excessively delaying it.
- Consume at least two, or preferably three, snacks a day; mid-morning and mid-afternoon are indispensable because they help buffer stomach acid, preventing it from rising too much due to prolonged fasting.

- Avoid a big dinner; it must always be quantitatively less than lunch.

- In general, it is good to limit binges because too abundant meals require a very extended gastric stay, strain the stomach, and need an acid secretion so significant as to cause discomfort to the already irritated mucosa.
- Chew slowly because correct and complete chewing makes digestion more comfortable, reducing food gastric residence time.
- Pay close attention to chewing the most stubborn or complicated foods (especially when the teeth do not allow it).
- It is advisable to remain in a sitting position for at least ten minutes after the meal.
- Cooking techniques that require a lot of fat: especially frying and those in a pan or pan with a lot of fat.

What to eat

- White meat (chicken, rabbit, turkey, veal)
- Cod, anchovies, sea bream, sea bass, tuna fillet, shrimp
- Wholemeal bread, White bread, Bread with cornflour, Brown rice, White rice, Pasta
- Lean ricotta, light spreadable cheese, Low-fat milk, Light yogurt, Mozzarella cheese
- Fruit with low citric acid content (e.g. apples, melons, pears, berries, bananas, peaches, etc.)
- Egg
- Fats of vegetable origin
- Vegetables: Carrots, Cabbage, Peas, Broccoli, Green Beans, Potatoes

The recommended cooking techniques are:

- Steam-powered
- In a pressure cooker
- Boil in water
- Baked
- Grilled
- In a skillet over low heat.

What to avoid

- Red meats
- Salmon, octopus, cuttlefish, mussels, clams, etc.
- Animal fats such as lard, bacon, hamburgers, pork fat cuts, hot dogs, etc.
- Onion and garlic
- Spices, Chili pepper
- Whole milk, Sour cream, Fatty cheeses, especially fermented ones
- Tomato
- Potato chips, candy or ice cream
- Foods preserved in salt, oil, smoked, etc
- Alcoholic drinks (especially spirits), tea, coffee, carbonated drinks
- Sour fruit (lemons, tangerines, oranges, pineapple, currants, pomegranates) and dried fruit (too rich in fat and protein), white wine, peppers, tomato juice, Vinegar
- Cocoa

The techniques not recommended are:

- Brazing
- Frying in a pan
- Stewing

Natural remedies

Natural remedies for gastritis aim on the one hand to reduce gastric secretion, and on the other hand to protect the mucous membrane of the stomach from the aggressiveness of acidic juices. Among the remedies that we can find in nature, we have:

CHAMOMILE

Its essential oil is used to relax the stomach muscles; thanks to this action, called antispasmodic, chamomile gives relief from cramps and abdominal pain. The habit of drinking a highly concentrated herbal tea based on chamomile is good prevention against the relapse of gastritis.

CABBAGE

Cabbage boasts healing properties for the digestive tract's mucous membranes: a glass of cabbage juice, combined with carrot and blueberry juice (which not only correct the taste but give it an excellent antioxidant power), could relieve gastritis.

CARROT

The carrot, rich in pectin - which can deposit itself as a sort of gel on the gastric walls, repairing them from the acid insult - contains another substance that protects the mucosa from attack by microorganisms: beta-carotene. Therefore, the precursor of vitamin A is classified as an excellent natural remedy against gastritis, also because it could promote the healing of any wounds (ulcer).

POTATO

The potato has emollient properties and calms the inflammation in the stomach, causing a pleasant sensation of relief.

LICORICE

It would be an excellent habit to chew bits of licorice to relieve the discomfort caused by gastritis. If the subject suffers from hypertension, licorice is not recommended because it favors the increase in blood pressure in high doses.

MAUVE

A mallow-based infusion is also useful if gastritis is associated with repeated abdominal cramps: mallow is an excellent natural remedy that relieves an irritated stomach.

GREEN TEA

In gastritis associated with ulcers, the essential constituents of tea are flavonoids, which stimulate healing.

SODIUM BICARBONATE

Further Advice

Bicarbonate is used to increase the stomach's pH and make the gastric environment less acidic; consequently, the burning sensation will be reduced, protecting the gastric mucosa from excessive acidity. It is advisable to dissolve a teaspoon of baking soda in a little water and drink it all. Sodium bicarbonate is contraindicated in case of hypertension and should never be taken together with too large meals.

- Drink more water: saliva and fluids protect the esophageal muscles from gastric juices.
- If gastritis symptoms are particularly intense and result in vomiting and/or diarrhea, it is essential to prevent dehydration by increasing the consumption of liquids: water or specific drinks that can be purchased at the pharmacy; instead, avoid coffee and sugary drinks.
- A walk at the end of the meal can help promote digestion.

- Out of respect for subjectivity, listen to your body and avoid the foods and drinks you attribute to past indigestion episodes. When the acute phase of gastritis has passed, experiment with ingesting small amounts of certain foods. Others may well tolerate some foods that are contraindicated for some and vice versa.
- In the acute phase, carefully follow the doctor's food recommendations; as soon as the symptoms subside, gradually expand the diet.

Chapter 4: Breakfast

1) Asparagus muffins

Ingredients:
- **Asparagus 380 g**
- **00 flour 250 g**
- **White yogurt 200 g**
- **Skimmed milk 200 g**
- **Eggs 120 g**
- **Parmesan 90 g**
- **Extra virgin olive oil 40 g**
- **Instant yeast for savory preparations 16 g**
- **Salt up to taste**
- **Basil to taste**

First, remove the toughest white part of the asparagus. Cut off the tips and cut the remainder of the stems into slices. Divide the tips in half lengthwise and keep them aside. Heat a little oil in a pan, add the asparagus slices and cook for 5 minutes over medium heat. After cooking, transfer the washers to a tall glass and blend with the hand blender to obtain a homogeneous puree. Now also place the pan's tips where you cooked the washers and sauté them for a few minutes, but they should not fall apart. Transfer the tips to a small bowl.

Take care of the dough: pour the eggs, olive oil, and milk into a bowl, then add salt. Stir with a hand whisk to mix and add the yogurt and yeast sifted through a colander. Stir in the sifted flour and mix again with a whisk. Season the mixture obtained with the grated cheese. Finish with the asparagus puree and some chopped basil leaves. Transfer the dough to a muffin mold. Do not fill the molds to the edge but leave a little margin to grow during cooking. Place the asparagus tips on the surface and cook in a preheated static oven at 200 ° for 20 minutes or until they are golden on the surface. When cooked, take the asparagus muffins out of the oven and let them cool before serving!

2) Potato plumcake

Ingredients:
- Potatoes 250 g
- 00 flour 200 g
- Skimmed milk at room temperature 100 g
- Eggs at room temperature 175 g
- Parmesan to grate 80 g
- Water at room temperature 50 g
- Instant yeast for savory preparations 16 g
- Thyme to taste
- Salt up to 4 g
- Extra virgin olive oil as needed
- Poppy seeds to taste

First, boil the potatoes for 30-40 minutes, until they are tender; cooking time may vary according to the potatoes' size. Once cooked, pass them still hot through the potato masher to reduce them to a puree. In a bowl, pour the flour, baking powder, and salt. Also, add the milk at room temperature. Continue pouring the water and eggs. Work with the electric whisk until the eggs are completely absorbed. At this point, add the cooled mashed potatoes and season with the thyme leaves and grated cheese. Mix and pour the dough into an oiled and floured plumcake mold, then level the surface with the back of the spoon. Grease a small knife with olive oil and then cut the dough's central part for the long side: this procedure will prevent the surface from splitting during cooking. Cover with poppy seeds and bake in a preheated static oven at 180 ° for 60 minutes on the central shelf. When cooked, take the potato plumcake out of the oven, let it cool and then turn it out to serve.

3) Savory donut with peas and ham

Ingredients:
- **Ricotta 140 g**
- **00 flour 140 g**
- **Skimmed milk 50 ml**
- **Medium eggs 3**
- **Seed oil 25 ml**
- **Peas 150 g**
- **Sliced raw ham 100 g**
- **Parmesan to grate 30 g**
- **Instant yeast for savory preparations 1 sachet**
- **Salt up to taste**
- **Extra virgin olive oil as needed**

In a pan, heat a drizzle of olive oil and add the peas. Stir in the water, add salt and lower the heat. Continue cooking for 10 minutes, stirring occasionally. Once ready, let it cool. Take the ham and cut it into strips. Keep aside. In a bowl, pour the eggs and milk, pour the seed oil, and mix everything with a hand whisk. Add the ricotta, a pinch of salt. Add the flour, the yeast for pies, and the grated Parmesan. Mix everything with a hand whisk. Stir in the peas and ham as well. Mix everything. Grease and flour a 24 cm diameter donut mold, pour the mixture inside, and level. Bake the donut in a preheated static oven at 180 ° for about 30 minutes. Let it cool, then unmold and serve.

4) Savory herb pancakes

Ingredients:
- Medium eggs 2
- 00 flour 100 g
- Skimmed milk 70 ml
- Swiss cheese 50 g
- 1 tbsp chopped chives
- Chopped parsley 2 tbsp
- Chopped basil 1 tbsp
- Instant yeast for savory preparations ½ tsp
- Salt up to taste
- Extra virgin olive oil (for the pan) 2 tbsp

FOR THE CREAM
- White yogurt 80 g
- 1 tbsp chopped chives
- Salt up to taste

Start grating the Swiss cheese coarsely and set it aside. Chop the herbs separately: chives, basil, and parsley. In a bowl, put the sifted flour and baking powder and add the grated cheese and one by one the chopped herbs: parsley, chives, and basil. In a separate bowl, beat the eggs with the milk and add the bowl's liquid containing the rest of the dry ingredients.

Mix well until the mixture is soft and homogeneous, add salt and stir for the last time. In a small non-stick pan, put 2 tablespoons of extra virgin olive oil and heat it on the stove: take 3 tablespoons of dough at a time and place them in a pan, which you will cook on both sides until golden. Remove the pancakes from the pan, drain them on absorbent paper and keep them warm; put another tablespoon of olive oil in the pan, and fry the remaining pancakes in the same way. Prepare the cream used to accompany the savory pancakes by mixing homogeneously, in a small bowl, the yogurt and half a tablespoon of chopped chives, and the salt. Serve the delicious herb pancakes with a tablespoon of cream on each and a sprinkling of leftover chives.

5) Yoghurt plum cake

Ingredients:
- 00 flour 300 g
- Eggs (about 5) 300 g
- Vegetable butter 200 g
- Low-fat yogurt 150 g
- Potato starch 50 g
- Powdered yeast 15 g
- Vanilla bean seeds 1
- Salt up to 4 g

First, put the vanilla pod's seeds, the diced butter, the flour, the eggs, the yogurt, the salt, the yeast, and the starch in a mixer. Work everything at maximum speed for about 3 and a half minutes. Meanwhile, grease and flour a loaf pan. As soon as you have obtained a homogeneous mixture, transfer it inside. Dip the blade of a knife, first in melted butter and then in the center of the plum cake. This will allow for uniform growth in cooking. Now take care of cooking the plumcake, which must be cooked in a preheated static oven in 2 phases: first at 185 ° for 15 minutes, then at 165 ° for 30 minutes. As soon as they are cooked, take them out of the oven and let them cool completely. At this point, turn them out, and the yogurt plumcakes are ready to taste.

6) Milk cake

Ingredients:
- **Skimmed milk 200 g**
- **Eggs 4**
- **00 flour 200 g**
- **Brown sugar 180 g**
- **Vegetable butter 60 g**
- **Powdered yeast for cakes 6 g**
- **Organic lemon zest 1**
- **Salt up to 1 pinch**

Break the eggs into a bowl, add a pinch of salt and operate the mixer. While the mixer is running, gradually add the sugar. When the mixture is clear and fluffy, about 10 minutes later, turn off the electric whisk. Place a colander over the bowl and sift the powders, then flour and yeast, adding them gradually while mixing with the spatula from the bottom to top. At this point, take a couple of spoonfuls of dough and set them aside in another container. In a saucepan, heat the milk over medium heat, then add the butter: let it melt entirely and bring everything just to touch the boil.

As soon as it reaches temperature, turn off the heat and pour the mixture into the container with the spoonfuls of dough that you had taken earlier. Mix well with a whisk to obtain a kind of batter. Now pour the batter into the larger container with the rest of the dough, mix gently with a spatula and finally grate the lemon zest. Grease and flour a 20 cm diameter cake pan and fill it with the mixture obtained. Bake in the static oven preheated to 180 ° on the lowest shelf for about 35 minutes. After the first 25 minutes, transfer the pan to the center shelf and continue for the remaining 10 minutes. As soon as the cake is ready, take it out of the oven and let it cool, remove it from the pan, and place it on a wire rack to cool completely. Your hot milk cake is ready to be enjoyed!

7) French brioches

Ingredients:
- **Warm skimmed milk 70 ml**
- **Fresh brewer's yeast 13 g**
- **Flour 0 550 g**
- **Vegetable softened butter 350 g**
- **Eggs 6**
- **Salt up to 15 g**
- **Brown sugar 80 g**
- **Yolks 1**

Start dissolving the brewer's yeast in warm milk; meanwhile, cut the butter into small pieces and let it soften at room temperature. In the bowl of a planetary mixer, mix the sifted flour, sugar, and salt. Add the yeast dissolved in milk and mix. Then add the eggs and mix for 6-8 minutes on a low speed. Increase the speed and add the softened butter one piece at a time, taking care to add the next when the previous one has been completely absorbed. Gradually the mixture will become frothy and light in color. Continue to add the butter and when you have obtained a very soft and homogeneous dough, put it in a bowl, cover it with plastic wrap and let it rise in the oven off with the light on for about 3 hours. After this time, knead the mixture again, turning the dough with your hand 2-3 times, and put it in the fridge, always covered with plastic wrap, for at least 12 hours, until the dough has solidified. The dough will now be remarkably compact: transfer it to a floured pastry board just enough to prevent the dough from sticking and roll it out into a 1 cm high sheet. Cut triangles of dough, roll them up to the tip on themselves. Curve the ends slightly inwards and place them on a dripping pan covered with parchment paper. Beat the egg yolk with milk in a small bowl and brush the brioches. Let them rise again for about 1 and 30 hours until they have doubled their volume. Bake the brioches in a preheated oven at 200 ° for 13-15 minutes, until they are golden on the surface. Here are your brioches ready to be enjoyed.

8) Muffin with Yogurt

Ingredients:
- **Flour 0 300 g**
- **Eggs 4**
- **Brown sugar 170 g**
- **Low-fat yogurt 220 g**
- **Salt up to 1 pinch**
- **Powdered yeast for cakes 16 g**
- **Soft vegetable butter 130 g**
- **Lemon zest 1**

First, make sure the butter is soft; leave it out of the fridge for about 30 minutes before using it. Then pour the butter into a planetary mixer equipped with a whisk (as an alternative to the planetary mixer, you can use an electric mixer), add the sugar and operate the machine by whipping the ingredients for at least 10 minutes at medium speed, until they have a consistency foamy. At this point, add the whole eggs, one at a time, taking care to wait until each egg is well incorporated before inserting another. Add the pinch of salt and the grated zest of 1 lemon. Finally, pour the yogurt a little and continue to whisk the dough until it is well blended. In a bowl, combine the yeast with the flour, incorporate the sifted powders into the dough through a sieve, mix with a spatula with movements from the bottom up. Now cut out 12 squares of parchment paper measuring 15x15 cm and line a mold of 12 muffins with these. Pour the mixture up to the edge of the mold. Once all the molds are filled, bake in a preheated static oven at 180 ° on the low shelf for 30 minutes or until they are golden on the surface. Once the yogurt muffins are ready, let them cool, then garnish them with the yogurt to taste and serve!

9) Pancakes without butter

Ingredients:
- Low-fat white yogurt 125 g
- 00 flour 150 g
- Skimmed milk 200 g
- Eggs 1
- Powdered yeast for cakes 8 g
- Extra virgin olive oil q.s.

Start by placing the egg in a bowl and beating it with a whisk. When it is light and fluffy, add the milk slowly and, continue to beat, add the yogurt. Then add, passing it through a sieve, the flour, and the baking powder. Proceed by mixing carefully, with gentle movements from the bottom to the top, to not disassemble the mixture, until you get a smooth and homogeneous batter. Cover with cling film, and place it in the fridge to rest for about 30 minutes. After this time, recover the batter and heat a non-stick pan with a drizzle of oil over medium heat.

Pour a spoonful of batter into the center of the pan, letting it spread by itself. After a few minutes, when small bubbles begin to bloom on the surface, it is time to turn the pancake with the help of a spatula. So cook it for another minute and when it's ready, place it on a plate. Continue like this until the batter is used up. Serve your butter-free pancakes with honey!

10) Apple biscuits

Ingredients:
- **Apples 200 g**
- **00 flour 250 g**
- **Yolks 2**
- **Salt up pinch 1**
- **Lemon zest 1**
- **Vegetable butter (cold from the fridge) 125 g**
- **Brown sugar 20 g**

Put the flour in a mixer and add the cold butter from the fridge cut into pieces. Run the mixer and let it work until you have obtained a sandy mixture, which you will transfer to a pastry board. Form the classic fountain, add the two egg yolks and a pinch of salt. Also, add the grated lemon zest and knead quickly, trying to heat the ingredients as little as possible until you get a compact dough. Cover the dough with a clean, dry cloth and let it rest. Meanwhile, cut the apples into slices and then into cubes of about half a centimeter in size. Roll out the pastry with a rolling pin and add the apple cubes, distributing them over the pastry's entire surface. Mix everything, trying to mix the apple cubes well into the pastry. Working it, the dough will heat up and become wetter, so add another 50 grams of flour to re-compact the dough as you knead it. Give your dough the shape of a sausage, then wrap it in cling film and let it rest in the refrigerator for an hour. After this time, remove the sausage from the fridge and unwind it from the film, placing it on a cutting board. With a knife, cut into discs 1 centimeter thick. With these doses, you will get about twenty. Pour the brown sugar into a bowl and gently press one side of each biscuit into the sugar so that the sugar grains adhere to the surface. Arrange the biscuits on the baking tray covered with parchment paper well spaced and bake in a preheated static oven at 180 ° for about 20-25 minutes, until the surface of the biscuits takes on color and the sugar has formed a light crust. When your cookies are cooked, take them out of the oven and let them cool before serving: your apple cookies are ready to be enjoyed!

11) Biscuits with olive oil

Ingredients:
- 00 flour 280 g
- Extra virgin olive oil ml
- Brown sugar 100 g
- Eggs 2
- Baking powder for cakes 10 g
- Salt up to 1 pinch
- Lemon zest 1
- Vanilla bean 1
- Yolks 1

Put the whole eggs plus the yolk in a bowl and beat with the sugar for a minute; then, continuing to beat, add the extra virgin olive oil and the aromas (the seeds of the vanilla pod and the lemon zest). Sift the flour and yeast in a bowl, add the salt, add the egg and sugar mixture and start kneading: when you have blended all the ingredients and obtained a smooth and homogeneous dough, wrap it in cling film and leave it to rest in the fridge to at least half an hour. After the indicated time, roll out the dough on a floured pastry board until it is half a centimeter thick, then make round shapes with a diameter of 5 cm, which you will place on a baking sheet lined with parchment paper and bake in a preheated static oven at 180 ° for about 15 minutes. Once cooked, take the cookies out of the oven, let them cool completely, and then store them in a tin box with a lid or an airtight container.

12) Gluten free sponge cake

Ingredients:
- **Eggs 5**
- **Brown sugar 150 g**
- **Vanilla bean 1**
- **Corn starch gluten free 150 g**

Start by placing the eggs in a planetary mixer, then add the sugar and whisk the ingredients for at least 10/15 minutes with a whisk until the mixture is frothy, puffy, and light yellow. If you wish, when the mixture is well whipped, you can add the seeds of the vanilla pod that you have cut in half and continue whipping for a few seconds to mix it well and flavor the mixture. At this point, you can add the starch (or potato starch) that you have previously well sieved: mix everything with a wooden spoon until you get a homogeneous mixture, being careful not to dismantle it. Grease and flour a round pan with a diameter of 24 cm with the starch, pour the dough into the mold's center, leveling it well. Bake the gluten-free sponge cake for about 35-40 minutes at 180 ° C in a preheated static oven without ever opening the oven in the first half-hour of cooking. Remove the mold from the oven and let the sponge cake cool in the mold before opening it.

Chapter 5: Appetizers, side dishes and snack

1) Watermelon and goat cheese finger food

Ingredients:

- **Watermelon baby variety 200 g**
- **Goat cheese 160 g**
- **Chives to taste**
- **Salt up to taste**
- **Extra virgin olive oil q.s.**

Start with the watermelon, then cut off the cap, make slices about 3 cm thick. For each slice, make cuts at a distance of about 3 cm from each other; do the same operation in the other direction to create cubes. Remove the peel and get your cubes; then, make a hollow in each cube with a small digger. In a bowl, pour the goat cheese and extra virgin olive oil, salt; add the chopped chives, taking the greenest and most fragrant part and work everything to mix. Once you have a homogeneous cream, stuff each cube with a tuft of goat cream, sprinkle with more chopped chives as you like, and serve your finger food!

2) Asparagus rolls

Ingredients:
- **Asparagus 16**
- **Phyllo dough 2 sheets**
- **Salt up to taste**

Take the asparagus, rinse them, dry them with a clean cloth, cut the white base, and remove the thinnest part of the stem with the vegetable peeler. In a pot full of boiling salted water, immerse them and let them cook for 5 minutes. When they are ready, drain them in a bowl of water and ice and leave them like this for a minute: in this way, cooking will stop, and the color will not fade. Now unroll the phyllo dough and use only two sheets, overlap them and cut with a knife; you will get 16 rectangles of the same size. Drain the asparagus and dry them well with absorbent paper, then arrange the asparagus in each of the rectangles of phyllo paper and wrap. Arrange parchment paper on the lined pan and continue like this with all the others. Bake them in a static oven, already hot at 200 °, for about 15 minutes, and they will be ready to be served

3) Rolls of zucchini and shrimp

Ingredients:
- Zucchini 160 g
- Shrimp 12 (clean)
- Breadcrumbs 80 g
- 1 sprig parsley
- Extra virgin olive oil 2 tbsp
- Salt up to taste

Wash it and trim the ends of the zucchini, then cut 12 skinny slices. Finally, chop the parsley, which you will need both for the flavored oil and bread. Pour the oil into a small bowl, add a teaspoon of chopped parsley and mix, brush the shrimp with the flavored oil, and add salt. To make the breading, pour the breadcrumbs into a bowl, add 2 tablespoons of chopped parsley, salt, and mix. Now you can assemble the rolls: place a slice of zucchini on a plate, place a shrimp at the lower end and roll it all up to the other end, then cover the roll obtained with the flavored breadcrumbs and transfer it to a baking tray lined with paper. oven. Continue in the same way with the rest of the ingredients when all the rolls are ready, season with a drizzle of oil and bake in a preheated static oven at 200 ° for 12 minutes. Once ready, serve your zucchini and shrimp rolls immediately!

4) Chia seed biscuits

Ingredients:
- **Eggs 8**
- **00 flour 250 g**
- **Vegetable butter 250 g**
- **Potato starch 125 g**
- **Parmesan to grate 125 g**
- **Chia seeds 80 g**

First, boil the eggs starting from cold water and cooking them for 8 minutes from the boil. Then drain them, let them cool and peel them. At this point, take only the yolks; the egg whites will not be used for this recipe. Cut the cold butter into cubes and place it in a mixer equipped with blades; add the flour, the starch, and blend everything until you get a crumbly mixture. Then add the Parmesan, the firm egg yolks, and the chia seeds. Blend everything again until the ingredients are combined. Then transfer the dough onto a lightly floured surface and knead it for a few minutes. Then wrap it in cling film. Let it rest in the refrigerator for at least 40 minutes. Then take the dough and roll it out on a surface with a little flour. You will need to obtain a thickness of 1 cm. Using a 5 cm diameter pastry cutter, cut the cookies and place them on a dripping pan lined with parchment paper. Bake in a preheated static oven at 180 °, on the low shelf for about 25/28 minutes, then take them out of the oven and let your chia seed biscuits cool before moving them to a tray.

5) Croutons of bread with rosemary lentil cream

Ingredients:
- Bay leaf 2 leaves
- Vegetable broth 400 ml
- Cloves 3
- Juniper berries 3
- Extra virgin olive oil 3 tbsp
- Salt up to taste
- Dried lentils 200 g

FOR 10 CROUTONS
- Vegetable Butter 80 g
- Baguette 10 slices
- 1 sprig rosemary

In a non-stick pan, fry the bay leaves, juniper berries, and cloves with a little oil over low heat. After 2 minutes, add the dried lentils. Cook everything for a few minutes, always over low heat; Wet the lentils with the broth, and continue cooking for at least 45/60 minutes, with the pot covered. Check often that the legumes do not dry out too much: in this case, add a few broth ladles. Once the lentils are ready, transfer them to a mixer, keep a little aside for the final garnish, reduce them to a cream, and then melt half of the butter provided in the recipe in a non-stick pan.

Add the lentil cream, chopped rosemary, and a little water to the melted butter to make the cream itself more fluid; mix everything, being careful not to let the mixture dry out too much. Slice the bread and melt the remaining butter in another pan, in which you will toast the croutons for a couple of minutes, turning them on both sides. Now transfer the lentil cream on each crouton, finally garnish with a little of the lentils that you had kept aside, with the help of a teaspoon and a few needles of rosemary.

6) Steamed aromatic meatballs

Ingredients:
- Minced veal 600 g
- Water 1.5 l
- Stale bread crumb 50 g
- Vegetable broth 50 ml
- Eggs 2
- Thyme 20 sprigs
- Laurel 3 leaves
- Chives 5 g
- Parsley 5 g
- Marjoram 5 g
- Salt up to taste

Start chopping the aromatic herbs: chop the chives, parsley, thyme, marjoram with a knife and set aside. Take the stale bread, remove the crust, cut the crumb into cubes, place it in a mixer, and chop finely. Take a large pot with a steaming basket and pour in the water, and add the bay leaf. Beat the eggs in a bowl, add salt. In another bowl, put the minced meat, the previously beaten eggs, and lastly, the crumb chopped with the mixer. Knead everything until the mixture is homogeneous and compact. : chives, parsley, thyme, marjoram. Now form the meatballs: try to get some meatballs of more or less the same size (weighing about 20 g each) to have homogeneous cooking. Stick the meatballs with toothpicks, heat the water in the pot, and wait for it to boil. Place the aromatic meatballs in the steamer and cook for about 18 minutes covered with the lid. (If you want, you can also cook the meatballs in the oven: place the meatballs in an oiled baking dish and cook in a static oven for 30 minutes at 180 ° or in a convection oven at 160 ° for about 25 minutes). Once cooked, serve the steamed aromatic meatballs hot; if you like, you can accompany them with a fresh salad.

7) Quinoa morsels

Ingredients:
- **Quinoa 150 g**
- **Small zucchini 2**
- **Eggs 1**
- **Parmesan to be grated 50 g**
- **Fresh ginger to grate to taste**
- **Salt up to taste**

Start by placing the quinoa in a bowl and rinsing it under cold water until the water is clear. Then boil the quinoa in a non-stick pan with salted water for the minutes indicated on the package (about 15-20 minutes), until the grains have absorbed most of the cooking water, softening and swelling. Proceed by draining the quinoa and passing it under cold water to stop cooking. At this point, carefully wash the zucchini and peel them. Then peel and clean the fresh ginger as well. Grate the zucchini and place them in a large bowl, and the fresh grated ginger. Add the boiled quinoa to the ginger's grated zucchini and add the grated Parmesan and the egg. Season with salt to taste and mix the ingredients until you get a homogeneous mixture. Proceed by placing the miniature paper cups (about 4-5 cm in diameter and about 3 cm high) on a baking sheet and fill them with the mixture; you can also use a non-stick mini muffin pan.

Compact the mix inside the cups with the back of a spoon to better define the morsels' shape. You just have to bake them in a preheated oven at 180 ° for 25 minutes (if you use a convection oven, cook them at 160 ° for 20 minutes) until the surface reaches a pleasant browning. At this point, the quinoa morsels are ready to be served and served warm!

8) Roast Potato Towers

Ingredients:
- **Rosemary to taste**
- **Extra virgin olive oil 12 tbsp**
- **Potatoes 5 (about 130 gr each)**
- **Salt to taste**

Carefully peel the potatoes, then cut them into relatively thin slices (about 3 mm). Be careful to cut the potatoes, keep them straight, and obtain slices that are as round and regular as possible. Finely chop the rosemary with a mixer and start composing the turrets: place salt on the first slice of potato, and a pinch of chopped rosemary, overlap a second slice, and season again with salt and rosemary: proceed in the same way until forming some "towers" about 4 cm high. When you have made them all, place them on a dripping pan covered with baking paper and pour a tablespoon of extra virgin olive oil on the surface of each turret. Bake everything at maximum power in your oven for 25-30 minutes until golden brown (be careful not to scorch the potatoes too much). The roasted potato towers are ready: serve hot.

9) Baked rice croquettes

Ingredients:
- Rice 500 g
- Extra virgin olive oil 30 g
- 1L vegetable broth

FOR BREADING
- Breadcrumbs 200 g
- Eggs (medium) 4
- Salt up to taste

FOR THE STUFFING:
- Raw ham 220 g
- Peas 180 g
- Mozzarella 150 g

Toast the rice for a few moments in the pot. Add the broth as the rice absorbs the liquids (this will take about 20 minutes). When cooked, turn off the heat. Transfer the risotto to a large pan and distribute it evenly with a spatula; cover the pan with plastic wrap and let it cool. Meanwhile, cut the ham into cubes. Steam the peas for 2 minutes and also cut the mozzarella into cubes. When the rice is cold, divide it into 26 portions of 50 g each; Take one, flatten it slightly with your hands giving it an oval shape, stuff the central part with the ham, the peas, and finally the mozzarella. Then close the croquettes with the rice giving them an elongated shape. Bread the croquettes, bypassing them first in the beaten egg and then in the breadcrumbs.

Repeat the same operation, proceeding to dip the already breaded croquette in the egg and then in the breadcrumbs. At this point, place the croquettes in a baking dish and sprinkle them with a drizzle of extra virgin olive oil. Bake in a preheated static oven at 200 ° C for 30-35 until the croquettes are golden brown. Serve the baked rice croquettes hot to preserve their crunchiness.

10) Baked Pumpkin flowers

Ingredients:
- Zucchini flowers 12
- Ricotta 400 g
- Oregano to taste
- Salt up to taste
- Extra virgin olive oil as needed
- Breadcrumbs 20 g
- Grated cheese 20 g

Pour the ricotta into a colander placed on a small bowl; sift the ricotta with the help of a spatula to make it finer. Flavored with oregano, finally salted. Then mix all the ingredients with a whisk. Now take care of cleaning the zucchini flowers: first, cut off the stem and remove the leaves from the flower base. To remove any earth residues, blow into the flower and gently wipe with a brush. Keep the internal pistil if it is still yellow; if it is too dark, it is advisable to remove it. Now you can stuff your zucchini flowers: pour the filling inside until they are almost filled and then close them on top, wrapping the tips to seal them.

Arrange the stuffed zucchini flowers on a baking tray lined with baking paper. In a small bowl, pour the grated cheese and breadcrumbs, mix to mix the breading. Now sprinkle the flowers with a drizzle of olive oil, then spread the breading with a spoon, and then pour in a drizzle of olive oil again. Cook the zucchini flowers in a preheated oven at 240 ° for 7-8 minutes. When cooked, take the zucchini flowers out of the oven and let them cool before enjoying them!

11) Baked potato balls

Ingredients:
- Potatoes 800 g
- Parmesan to grate 40 g
- Breadcrumbs 60 g
- Eggs 1
- Parsley 1 bunch
- Oregano 4 leaves
- Dried thyme q.s.
- Salt up to taste

FOR BREADING
- Breadcrumbs 120 g
- Eggs 2
- Extra virgin olive oil 2 tbsp

First, boil the potatoes for 30-40 minutes. Chop the parsley after washing and drying it. Pass the potatoes while still hot with their skin in a potato masher and collect the puree in a bowl. Add the salt, pepper, thyme, grated Parmesan, a few oregano leaves, and the chopped parsley. Mix everything well, then add the egg and breadcrumbs. Mix to obtain a homogeneous mixture. Now make meatballs by lightly squeezing them with your hands and transfer them to a tray. Prepare the breading: In a bowl, beat the eggs; in another dish, pour the breadcrumbs. Then take the meatballs, pass them in the egg, and then in the breadcrumbs.

Transfer all the meatballs to a baking sheet covered with parchment paper, season with 2 tablespoons of oil, and bake in a preheated oven at 180 ° C for 15 minutes or until golden brown. After the cooking time, take the baked potato balls out of the oven and serve hot!

12) Breaded sandwich

Ingredients:
- **Mozzarella 200 g**
- **Eggs 2**
- **Salt up to taste**
- **Loaf bread 140 g (8 slices)**
- **Skimmed milk 50 g**
- **Breadcrumbs to taste**

Cut off the edges of the bread, then cut the mozzarella into slices. The mozzarella must be well dried so that it does not lose any liquid during cooking. In a separate bowl, beat the salted eggs. Take a slice of bread, lay the slices of mozzarella on top, and then close like a sandwich with another slice. Pour the milk into a bowl and dip the sandwich inside, then pass it in the beaten eggs and then finish the breading with the breadcrumbs, carefully covering the surface and edges of the bread. It is possible to proceed with cooking: line a baking tray with parchment paper and place the pieces to be cooked; cook in a preheated oven at 200 ° for 15 minutes in static mode. When cooked, take the pan out of the oven and serve hot and stringy.

Chapter 6: Fish and Seafood

1) Salad rolls stuffed with tuna

Ingredients:
- **Tuna fillet 100 g**
- **Lettuce 4 leaves**
- **Broad beans 400 g**
- **Extra virgin olive oil 40 g**
- **Basil 3 leaves**
- **Salt up to taste**
- **Low-fat yogurt 20 g**
- **Chopped pistachios to taste**
- **Chives 8 strands**

Shell the beans and collect them in the mixer's glass, pour the olive oil, and blend to obtain a cream. Also, add the yogurt, salt, and mix with a spoon to combine. Scent, the cream with the chopped basil, leaves with your hands. In a pan with a drizzle of oil, brown the tuna for a few minutes. Now take the lettuce leaves, wash them well under running water, then dry them thoroughly with a cloth. Divide each leaf in half, taking care to remove the more rigid central core. Take one half of the lettuce leaf, spread the cream of beans and yogurt, and the entire leaf and stuff with the cooked tuna cut into chunks.

Roll up the leaf, tie it with a thread of chives to seal the roll. Garnish with chopped pistachios to taste and continue in the same way for all the others. Your salad rolls stuffed with tuna are ready to be brought to the table. Accompany them with an extra cream of broad beans!

2) Cod with yogurt and purple potatoes

Ingredients;
- **Cod 400 g**
- **Natural white yogurt 120 g**
- **Purple potatoes 200 g**
- **Extra virgin olive oil 60 g**
- **Salt up to taste**
- **Thyme to taste**
- **4 slices bread**
- **Vegetable butter 40 g**

Take the cod fillets, and boil them in a pot for about 10 minutes, until they are white and tender. Pour the potatoes into cold water and cook for about 15 minutes from boiling. Then drain and peel them. In a blender, pour the cod and purple potatoes, peeled and coarsely cut into pieces, add the extra virgin olive oil, season with salt and start blending everything. Keep running the mixer while adding the white yogurt, then work until you get a smooth and whipped cream. Add the thyme leaves.

Transfer the mixture to the fridge for at least 10-15 minutes. Cut 4 slices of bread, then take the butter and spread it on the bread, then arrange them on a dripping pan lined with baking paper and toast the slices in a static oven preheated to 200 ° for about 10 minutes, until they are golden brown. Serve your creamy cod mousse with yogurt and purple potatoes on the toasted bread, and add a few thyme leaves.

3) Tuna cheesecake

Ingredients:
- **Natural tuna fillets 200 g**
- **Light spreadable cheese 200 g**
- **Bread crumbs 100 g**
- **Vegetable butter 120 g**
- **Extra virgin olive oil 30 g**
- **Chives a few stems**
- **Salt up to taste**

Place the bread crumbs in the mixer and blend them to obtain crumbs. Heat a non-stick pan, pour in the bread crumbs, and toast them for a few minutes until golden. Now melt the butter in the microwave or a bain-marie, pour it over the bread crumbs, stir to mix, and pour a couple of tablespoons of crumbs into a 9 cm diameter pastry ring. Press the base well with the back of a spoon. Put the base to harden in the refrigerator for at least 15 minutes. In the meantime, prepare the cream: pour the cheese, tuna, and chives into the mixer, add salt, add the olive oil and blend everything to obtain a homogeneous cream. Once the base has firmed, completely cover the bread with the cream, and level the surface with the back of a teaspoon. Put back in the refrigerator to harden for 10 minutes. Once the cream has also firmed up, take the cheesecakes, garnish them with a few tuna pieces, and finally flavored with chives. The tuna cheesecake is ready to serve.

4) Cod and ham morsels

Ingredients:
- **Cod fillet 300 g**
- **Sliced raw ham 100 g**
- **Bread (crumb) 30 g**
- **1 sprig rosemary**
- **1 sprig parsley**
- **Chives to taste**
- **Salt up to 1 pinch**
- **Extra virgin olive oil as needed**

First, prepare the chopped herbs and add them to a bowl together with the crumbled breadcrumbs. Take the cod fillets and cut them into cubes, not too small. Pour a drizzle of oil into a pan, heat it, and add the cod. Let it brown on both sides for a total of 5 minutes, turning them gently. Finally, add salt and transfer to a plate. Then pass the cod cubes in the breading to cover them entirely. Spread the slices of ham on a cutting board and place each codpiece at the beginning of one of the slices. Roll up to obtain a roll. Do the same for the others and place them in an ovenproof dish. Bake in a preheated static oven at 180 ° for 10 minutes. Then remove from the oven and let it cool. Arrange some lettuce leaves and a small bowl on a plate, then transfer the morsels as well. Your cod bites are ready to serve!

5) Honey roasted shrimp

Ingredients:
- Shrimp (Clean) 36
- Honey 100 g
- Fresh ginger 3 g
- Salt up to taste

FOR THE FAKE MAYONNAISE
- Sunflower oil 100 ml
- Soy milk 50 ml
- Mint 8 leaves
- Salt up to taste

Peel and grate the fresh ginger. Pour the honey into a saucepan and the ginger and salt 8. Heat and thicken by cooking over moderate heat for 5 minutes. Then let the sauce cool. Now compose the skewers: skewer 3 shrimp on each wooden skewer. Set aside and prepare the fake mayonnaise: pour the seed oil, milk, and mint leaves into a tall, narrow bowl. Add salt and blend with the immersion blender until you get a smooth cream. You can then proceed with cooking, brush the skewers with the honey sauce, and then cook on a hot grill on both sides for a couple of minutes. Serve the skewers roasted with honey accompanying them with the fake mint mayonnaise.

6) Sole in the pan

Ingredients:
- **Clarified butter 120 g**
- **00 flour q.s.**
- **1 sprig parsley**
- **Salt up to taste**
- **Skimmed milk to taste**
- **Medium sole 4 (clean)**

Dip the sole in the milk and then pass them in the flour on both sides. Then place them in a pan with the clarified butter, cooking them for 3-4 minutes on each side until they are golden brown on each side: be very careful not to break the soles when you turn them! Meanwhile, chop the parsley with a knife. When the sole is ready, add salt and sprinkle with chopped parsley. Serve the sole immediately, decorating the dish with sprigs of parsley!

7) Tuna with sesame

Ingredients:
- **Tuna (4 fillets) 150 g**
- **Black sesame seeds 10 g**
- **White sesame seeds 20 g**
- **Extra virgin olive oil 35 g**
- **Lemon juice 25 g**
- **Salt up to taste**

In a dish, pour the sesame seeds, and mix them. Take the tuna: we recommend that you make sure that the tuna you have purchased has been slaughtered; however, we recommend that you freeze it for at least 96 hours at -18 degrees, then defrost it before using the recipe. Pass the slices of tuna over the seeds to bread them on both sides as evenly as possible. Heat a non-stick pan and only when it is hot, place the breaded tuna fillets and cook over high heat for 1 minute, then turn them with a spatula, continue cooking for another minute. Once seared, the tuna will be raw inside, but you can extend the cooking according to your taste if you like. Once cooked, transfer the fillets to a cutting board, immediately cut them into slices, and serve immediately.

8) Sea bream with carrots and zucchini

Ingredients:
- **Sea bream 2 pieces (clean)**
- **Extra virgin olive oil 30 g**
- **Carrots 150 g**
- **Zucchini 150 g**
- **Thyme to taste**

Wash and peel the carrots, then trim the ends and cut them into slices of about 5 mm thick. Wash and trim the zucchini, too, cut them in half lengthwise and then further divide each half; finally, cut them into cubes of about 1 cm thick. Pour the oil into a large non-stick pan and when it is hot, place the sea bream inside, then add the carrots, the zucchini, the spring onion, and the sprigs of thyme, and add salt. Cover the pan with a lid and cook over medium heat for 7 minutes, then turn the sea bream with the help of 2 spatulas, being careful not to break them; cover again with the lid and cook for another 7 minutes. Of course, cooking times may vary depending on the weight of the sea bream you will use. The pan-fried sea bream is ready to be served!

9) Cod fillet with pistachio pesto

Ingredients:
- **Cod fillets 2**
- **Extra virgin olive oil q.s.**
- **Salt up to taste**

FOR THE PISTACHIO PESTO
- **Unsalted pistachios 30 g**
- **Extra virgin olive oil 30 g**
- **Salt up to taste**

Pour the shelled pistachios into a blender, add the oil and a pinch of salt, and blend until a smooth cream is obtained, then transfer the pistachio pesto into a bowl and set aside. Heat a little oil in a non-stick pan, add the cod fillets, add salt and cook over medium-high heat for 2-3 minutes. At this point, gently turn the fillets with a spatula and cook them on the other side for 1-2 minutes, then remove them from the pan. Spread a spoonful of pistachio pesto on each plate, place the cod fillet. Your cod fillet with pistachio pesto is ready to serve!

10) Swordfish and broccoli medallions

Ingredients:
- **Swordfish fillet 400 g**
- **Broccoli 200 g**
- **Potatoes 400 g**
- **Marjoram 3 sprigs**
- **Extra virgin olive oil q.s.**
- **Salt up to taste**

Put two pans with water to bring to the boil; in one place, the thoroughly washed potatoes when the water is still cold, when it boils, calculate for about 30-40 minutes. Meanwhile, wash the broccoli, put them in the other pan when the water has boiled, and simmer for about 5 minutes. Then drain the broccoli and chop coarsely with a knife, then let them cool. When the potatoes are cooked, peel and mash them with a potato masher in a large bowl, then preheat the oven to 200 ° in static mode. Finally, take the swordfish fillets, cut them into cubes, and then chop them coarsely with a knife. When the vegetables have cooled, take the bowl where you mashed the potatoes, add the chopped broccoli and swordfish, salt, and add the marjoram leaves, then mix with your hands to mix all the ingredients.

Take some dough and shape it with a 6.5 cm diameter pastry ring to form the medallions: with these doses, you should get 6. Transfer the medallions on a baking tray lined with parchment paper, season with a drizzle of oil, then bake them in a preheated static oven at 200° for about 20 minutes. After the medallions' cooking time, take them out of the oven and transfer them to a serving dish, add a few leaves of marjoram, and season with a drizzle of raw oil. Your cod and broccoli medallions are ready to be served!

11) Tuna steak with mint pesto

Ingredients:
- Tuna (a fresh fillet) 600 g

FOR MARINATING
- Extra virgin olive oil 10 g
- Chives to chop 1 tbsp
- Salt up to taste

FOR THE MINT PESTO
- Mint 20 g
- Extra virgin olive oil 100 ml
- Pine nuts 20 g
- Salt up to taste

Start by preparing the mint pesto: pour the well washed and dried mint leaves into the bowl of a mixer, add the pine nuts and olive oil. Add salt and use the mixer to obtain a homogeneous sauce. Now take care of the marinade: chop the chives in a bowl, pour the olive oil and chives. Place the tuna, massage it with the marinade on both sides. Leave to marinate for half an hour. Now go to cooking: Heat a non-stick pan well, place the tuna, and sear it for a minute on each side. Once cooked, cut the tuna into 2 cm thick slices. Place the tuna slices on a plate, season them with coarse salt and accompany your tuna steak with the mint pesto.

12) Mediterranean sea bass

Ingredients:
- **2 sea bass fillets**
- **Extra virgin olive oil 30 g**
- **Pitted black olives 50 g**
- **Pine nuts 20 g**
- **Thyme 2 sprigs**
- **Salt up to taste**

Put a pan with the oil on the heat, place the sea bass fillets. Cook for 2 minutes over medium heat; take care to turn them with a spatula halfway through cooking; do this very gently not to break the sea bass. At this point, add the olives. Salt and flavor the sea bass fillets with fresh thyme leaves. Turn off the heat and separately in another pan, toast the pine nuts for 2-3 minutes over medium heat. Serve the sea bass fillet with olives and garnish with toasted pine nuts!

Chapter 7: Meat

1) Salad baskets with turkey

Ingredients:
- **Turkey breast 250 g**
- **Baby lettuce 100 g**
- **Cashews 25 g**
- **Carrots 1**
- **Parsley to taste**
- **Extra virgin olive oil q.s.**

Place the turkey breast on a cutting board and cut it into irregular pieces. Then take a non-stick pan, heat a drizzle of oil. Add the turkey breast bites and salt. Cook the morsels for about 10 minutes, turning them from time to time to cook them inside until they are golden brown. When the turkey morsels are cooked, transfer them to a mixer, operate for a few seconds until the meat is well chopped, and then transfer the blended mixture into a large bowl. At this point, place the cashews on a cutting board and chop them coarsely. Sauté the chopped cashews in a non-stick pan and toast them for a few minutes, until crisp and darker. Then add the toasted cashews to the chopped turkey bites. Then take a carrot, peel it and divide it in half. After that, slice it into tiny cubes.

Also, wash the parsley under running water and chop finely on a cutting board. At this point, add the diced carrot and chopped parsley to the mixture. Now wash the salad carefully and leaf it through, placing the crispest and most curved leaves on a serving dish. Then proceed to fill them with the dough. Your baskets of lettuce with turkey are ready to be served.

2) Meatballs in sesame crust

Ingredients:
- **Minced veal 300 g**
- **Wholemeal bread crumb 65 g**
- **Parmesan (for grating) 50 g**
- **Sesame seeds 50 g**
- **Black sesame seeds 25 g**
- **Eggs 1**
- **Salt up to taste**

Cut the wholemeal bread crumb into cubes, removing the outer crust, and crumble it in a mixer. In a large bowl, pour the veal, mixing them with your hands; add the chopped breadcrumbs, then the grated cheese. Incorporate the egg and season with salt. Mix with your hands until you get a homogeneous mixture. Each and continue like this until you finish the mix available: with our doses, you will have to obtain 38 meatballs. Pour the white sesame seeds into a tray and add them to the black sesame seeds, mixing them carefully. Pass the meatballs over the sesame, making it stick well to the meat. Continue in this way with all the remaining meatballs and, once finished, arrange them side by side on a baking tray lined with baking paper. Bake the meatballs in a preheated static oven at 180 ° for about 25 minutes, seasoning them with a drizzle of oil if necessary. After the required time, take out of the oven and enjoy your sesame-crusted meatballs hot.

3) Veal slices with mushrooms

Ingredients:
- **Veal (walnut) 400 g**
- **Champignon mushrooms 500 g**
- **Vegetable butter 50 g**
- **00 flour 40 g**
- **Extra virgin olive oil 10 g**
- **Salt up to taste**
- **Thyme to taste**
- **1 sprig chopped rosemary**

Take the veal slices, and with the meat mallet, slice them to make them thinner, flour the veal slices on both sides, and then shake them to remove the excess flour. Now take care of cleaning the mushrooms: with a small knife, begin to remove the earthy part on the stem, scraping it gently until any traces of earth are removed. If the mushroom is clean enough, remove the few earth residues with a brush, do not wash them with water to not spoil them. Slice the mushrooms and set them aside. Now proceed with cooking the meat: In a pan, melt half a dose of butter (25 g), adding the olive oil; once melted, lay the floured veal slices, add salt and brown them for 3 minutes per side or until a crust forms.

Once golden brown, let them cool on a plate and take care of the mushrooms: In the same pan in which you cooked the meat, melt the other half of the butter, season with the chopped rosemary, add the sliced mushrooms and sauté over medium heat for two minutes. , then add salt. At this point, add the veal slices browned and kept aside and flavored with the thyme leaves, cook over low heat for a minute, adding a ladle of water if necessary, and serve the veal with the mushrooms very hot!

4) Milk chicken breasts

Ingredients:
- **Sliced chicken breast 4**
- **Vegetable butter 40 g**
- **Extra virgin olive oil 10 g**
- **00 flour q.s.**
- **Skimmed milk 170 g**
- **Salt up to taste**
- **Thyme 4 sprigs**

Arrange the slices on a cutting board and, using a meat mallet, beat them to obtain thin slices. Arrange the oil and butter in a pan, let it melt gently, and in the meantime, flour the chicken slices. As you move them into the pan, raise the heat slightly and wait about 2 minutes until a nice crust has formed. Then turn the slices, wait a couple of minutes again, pour the milk first, and then the thyme leaves into the pan. Add salt, cover with a lid and let it cook for another 4-5 minutes until the milk has thickened. At this point, you just have to serve your milk-filled chicken breasts still hot!

5) Tasty chicken wings and potatoes

Ingredients:
- Chicken wings 8
- Potatoes 500 g
- Breadcrumbs 200 g
- 00 flour 50 g
- Parmesan to grate 50 g
- Eggs 2
- Parsley to be minced to taste
- Extra virgin olive oil as needed
- Salt up to taste

First, pour the flour into a bowl and flour the chicken wings on both sides, remove the excess flour and place them on a tray. In another bowl, pour the breadcrumbs, grated Parmesan cheese, chopped parsley (keep some aside for the final garnish) and mix thoroughly. Finally, beat the eggs in another bowl again. Dip the floured chicken wings first in the beaten egg and then in the breadcrumbs and Parmesan cheese, pressing with your hands so that it adheres well. It is important to flour the meat first to prevent the breading from coming off during cooking. Once you have breaded all the chicken wings, you can take care of the potatoes. Peel the potatoes, divide them first in half and then in quarters, finally cut them into cubes. Put the potatoes in a bowl, season them with oil and salt, and then pour them into the bowl with the leftover breading and mix well. At this point, take a large pan and place the breaded chicken wings inside, then add the potatoes and distribute them evenly on the surface. Season with a little salt and a generous round of oil and cook in a preheated convection oven at 200 ° for 40 minutes. After this time, turn on the grill and continue cooking for another 10 minutes to make the breading crispy. Once cooked, garnish with the remaining parsley and serve your flavorful chicken wings and potatoes still steaming!

6) Stuffed turkey rolls

Ingredients:
- **Turkey breast (4 slices)**
- **Salt up to taste**
- **Seed oil 3 tbsp**
- **Rosemary 8 sprigs**
- **Scamorza 8 slices**
- **8 slices raw ham**

Beat the slices with a meat tenderizer, wrapping them with baking paper. Take a slice of chicken and stuff it first with 2 slices of smoked cheese and then with two slices of raw ham, roll the slice on itself. Cut the roll in half that you are going to stop with a wooden skewer. Flavor each roll with a sprig of rosemary. Proceed in the same way with all the other turkey slices. Now the rolls are ready for cooking: heat a grill brushed with a little seed oil, cook the rolls on both sides, at least 6/7 minutes per side until they are well grilled, finally add salt and let them rest before serving.

7) Roasted rabbit

Ingredients:
- **Rabbit in pieces 1.2 kg**
- **Rosemary 4 sprigs**
- **Salt up to taste**
- **Vegetable broth 2000 g**
- **Potatoes 800 g**
- **Thyme 4 sprigs**
- **Bay leaf 1 leaf**
- **Extra virgin olive oil 80 g**

Chop the rosemary, then transfer half of it into a pan where you have poured 40 g of oil. Add a bay leaf and let it cook over low heat for 2-3 minutes. Raise the heat, and add the rabbit pieces; let them brown on both sides for 3-4 minutes. Add a ladle of broth and cook over low heat for another 5-6 minutes. In the meantime, prepare the potatoes: peel them and cut them into rather large chunks. Transfer everything to a bowl, flavor with the chopped rosemary needles, and set aside the thyme leaves and salt. Drizzle with 20 g of oil and mix. Transfer everything to a large pan, oiled with about 10 g of oil, so that the potatoes are well distributed. Then also arrange the previously browned rabbit pieces. Add the remaining vegetable broth and cook the rabbit with the potatoes in a preheated static oven at 200 ° for 40 minutes. Once out of the oven, serve your rabbit in the oven while still steaming!

8) Chicken meatloaf

Ingredients:
- **Minced chicken 800 g**
- **Swiss cheese 150 g**
- **Ricotta 100 g**
- **Parmesan to grate 50 g**
- **Eggs 1**
- **Breadcrumbs 70 g**
- **Marjoram 3 sprigs**
- **Extra virgin olive oil 10 g**
- **Salt up to taste**

First, cut the cheese into cubes, then transfer them to a blender and blend everything. Transfer to a bowl with the minced chicken, then add the well-drained ricotta, grated cheese, marjoram leaves, salt, and egg. Knead with your hands to mix the ingredients, then add the breadcrumbs and knead again until the mixture is smooth. Pour the mixture onto a sheet of parchment paper and shape it with your hands to give it the shape of meatloaf, then wrap it in the same parchment paper and seal the roll. Leave to harden in the refrigerator for at least an hour. After this time, remove the parchment paper and heat the oil in a pan or a large pot suitable for cooking in the oven. Brown the meatloaf on all sides so that it forms a nice crust, using two stirrers or kitchen tongs to keep it from breaking. At this point, cover the pan with aluminum foil and bake at 200 ° in static mode for 60 minutes. Once cooked (if you have a thermometer, check that the internal temperature has reached 70 ° -71 °), take your chicken meatloaf out of the oven and serve it sprinkled with its cooking juices.

9) Turkey chunks with saffron

Ingredients:
- Turkey breast 600 g
- Saffron (one sachet) 0.15 g
- Water about 140 g
- Extra virgin olive oil 10 g
- Potato starch 1 tsp
- 00 flour q.s.
- Salt up to taste

FOR THE ASPARAGUS
- Asparagus 400 g
- Water 100 g
- Extra virgin olive oil 10 g
- Salt up to taste

Start by cleaning the asparagus: wash them, dry them, remove the toughest end, cut them diagonally, and keep them aside. Heat the oil in a pan, add the asparagus, add salt and cook over medium heat for 7-8 minutes, adding about 100 g of water to keep the vegetables from drying out. Once they are cooked, keep them aside and take care of the turkey. Cut the turkey breast into strips and then cut them into cubes of about 1.5-2 cm. Heat a little oil in a pan. Meanwhile, flour the diced turkey in a sieve so as to remove the excess flour. Once the oil is hot, add the turkey, let it brown and then wet with about 100 g of water, or just enough to keep the turkey from drying out. Dissolve the saffron in a little warm water and add it to the preparation; add salt, stir and continue cooking; the morsels must cook in total for about 10 minutes; the time may vary according to their size. Make a cream to thicken the preparation: pour a teaspoon of starch into a small bowl, dilute it with a couple of tablespoons of water and mix to obtain a homogeneous mixture. Add the melted starch to the still hot preparation and mix. Your chicken nuggets with saffron are ready; serve them accompanied with a side of asparagus.

10) Chicken strips with radicchio

Ingredients:
- **Chicken breast 650 g**
- **400 g long radicchio**
- **Brown sugar 30 g**
- **Water 100 g**
- **Extra virgin olive oil 10 g**

FOR MARINATING
- **Extra virgin olive oil 50 g**
- **Thyme 2 sprigs**
- **Marjoram 2 sprigs**
- **Salt up to taste**

Take the chicken breast, cut it in half, and make some pretty thin strips. Pour the oil into a pan, add the thyme and marjoram leaves, and season with salt. Distribute the strips of chicken next to each other in the pan so that the marinade is evenly distributed; cover with cling film and refrigerate for at least 2 hours. Wash the radicchio with plenty of fresh running water; remove the base, cut it in half, remove the hard edge, and then cut it into strips lengthwise. In a pan, add the water, the brown sugar and cook for another 2 minutes. Also, add the radicchio cut into strips and cook for 2 minutes, raising the heat. Remove the chicken from the refrigerator and add it to the vegetables. Cook for 2-3 minutes and, when the chicken turns brown, turn off. Finally, you can serve and taste your chicken strips with radicchio.

11) Veal skewers with rocket and scamorza cheese

Ingredients:
- Slices of veal 600 g
- Scamorza 200 g
- Rocket 50 g
- Extra virgin olive oil q.s.
- Salt up to taste

Detach the rocket leaves from the stem, wash them under running water, and then pat them with a kitchen towel to dry them. Cut the scamorza cheese into thin slices, then beat the veal slices between two sheets of paper. Spread one of the slices of meat on the cutting board, place the slices of smoked cheese on top and cover with the rocket. Roll the meat lengthwise to form a roll. Now insert some skewers inside, which will hold the filling in place and facilitate cutting. Divide the veal roll into 4 parts, gently remove the skewers and reinsert them inside each part. Heat a pan with a few tablespoons of extra virgin olive oil and place the veal skewers inside. Cook them for 7 minutes, turning them halfway through cooking. Add salt and serve your veal skewers with rocket and scamorza.

12) Loin of rabbit mashed carrots

Ingredients:
- **12 rabbit loins**
- **5 carrots**
- **Vegetable broth 2 spoon**
- **Oil**
- **Salt**
- **Vegetable butter 1 teaspoon**

Heat three tablespoons of oil, add the diced carrots and two tablespoons of broth, cook, and add salt. Remove and blend until you have a smooth cream. Heat four tablespoons of oil and a knob of butter, place the rabbit loins in it, brown them evenly, salt them at the end. Remove them and cut each loin into two or three pieces. On the bottom of the serving dish, pour the carrot purée and, on top, the rabbit loins. Serve.

Chapter 8: Unique dishes

1) Lentil pie

Ingredients:
- **Potatoes 400 g**
- **Lentils 100 g**
- **Spinach 400 g**
- **Eggs 1**
- **Mozzarella 50 g**
- **Parmesan 50 g**
- **Breadcrumbs 40 g**
- **Vegetable butter 50 g**
- **Extra virgin olive oil 30 g**
- **Salt up to taste**

First, wash the spinach. In a large pan, heat the oil, add the still moist spinach, add salt and cook for about 5 minutes, moving them with a wooden spoon. Finally, remove from the heat, and drain. Peel the potatoes and cut them into cubes. Pour the potatoes into a saucepan with boiling water. Rinse the lentils, drain them, and add them to the pot with the potatoes. Add salt and cook for about 20 minutes with the lid on. Finally, drain the vegetables and put them in a bowl. Mash with a fork until the potatoes and lentils are reduced to a creamy puree. Add 30 g of butter and mix. Also, add the Parmesan, stir again, and then add the egg as well. Mix well.

Cut the mozzarella into cubes. Grease 8 disposable aluminum molds with 10 g of melted butter with a pastry brush and sprinkle them with breadcrumbs. Fill each mold halfway with the mashed potatoes and lentils. Add a little cooked spinach and continue with or diced mozzarella. Finally, cover with the mixture of lentils and potatoes, pressing with the back of the spoon. Sprinkle with plenty of breadcrumbs. Put a small piece of butter on the surface and bake on the oven's middle shelf preheated to 180 ° C in static mode for about 30 minutes. Remove the golden pies from the oven, turn them out, and serve them still hot

2) Baskets of potatoes with zucchini and cheese

Ingredients:
- **Potatoes 300 g**
- **Zucchini 200 g**
- **Mozzarella g**
- **Extra virgin olive oil as needed**
- **Salt up to taste**
- **Oregano to taste**

Peel the potatoes and then cut them into 1 mm thin slices. Transfer them to a bowl and season with olive oil, salt, and oregano. Stir to flavor well and then butter 12 aluminum molds; arrange the potato slices first on the bottom and then on the inner edges to completely cover the molds. Now place them on an oven rack and cook in a preheated convection oven at 200 ° for 20 minutes. Meanwhile, cut the mozzarella into cubes, wash and trim the zucchini, then cut them into cubes. In a pan, pour the oil and add the zucchini, add salt and cook for 15 minutes over medium heat. After cooking, keep aside. Meanwhile the baskets will have finished cooking, take them out of the oven. Stuff the baskets with a few cubes of mozzarella, then with the zucchini, and finish with a last layer of mozzarella. At this point, put it back in the oven for 10 minutes, just long enough to melt the mozzarella. Turn out the potato baskets, let them cool slightly, and then serve them on the table.

3) Chickpea crepes with cod mousse

Ingredients

- **Chickpea flour 100 g**
- **Water 250 g**
- **Extra virgin olive oil 1 tbsp**
- **Salt up to 1 pinch**

FOR THE COD MOUSSE
- **Cod 600 g**
- **Skimmed milk 300 g**
- **Ricotta 100 g**
- **Sage 1 leaf**
- **Bay leaf 1 leaf**
- **Parsley 5 g**
- **Chives to taste**
- **Salt up to 1 pinch**

Peel the potatoes and then cut them into 1 mm thin slices. Transfer them to a bowl and season with olive oil, salt, and oregano. Stir to flavor well and then butter 12 aluminum molds; arrange the potato slices first on the bottom and then on the inner edges to completely cover the molds. Now place them on an oven rack and cook in a preheated convection oven at 200 ° for 20 minutes. Meanwhile, cut the mozzarella into cubes, wash and trim the zucchini, then cut them into cubes. In a pan, pour the oil and add the zucchini, add salt and cook for 15 minutes over medium heat. After cooking, keep aside. Meanwhile, the baskets will have finished cooking, take them out of the oven. Stuff the baskets with a few cubes of mozzarella, then with the zucchini, and finish with a last layer of mozzarella. At this point, put it back in the oven for 10 minutes, just long enough to melt the mozzarella. Turn out the potato baskets, let them cool slightly, and then serve them on the table.

4) Shrimp omelette

Ingredients:
- **Medium eggs 8**
- **Shrimp 800 g (Clean)**
- **Parsley 4 sprigs**
- **Extra virgin olive oil 20 g**
- **Salt up to taste**

Wash the parsley stalks and pat them dry with a clean kitchen towel or paper towel. Then place them on a cutting board and chop finely. At this point, break the eggs into a bowl, beat them with a fork or whisk, and add salt to taste. Take a non-stick pan, heat the oil and pour the parsley and fry for a few seconds. Pour the cleaned and shelled prawns into the sauce and brown them over medium heat for about 5 minutes, until they are slightly pink. After this time, add the beaten eggs to the pan, tilting the pan to ensure that the mixture covers the pan's entire surface. Let it cook for 2 minutes over low heat, then cover with a lid and continue to cook for 5-6 minutes, until the surface is sufficiently thickened. At this point, turn the omelet with the help of the lid or a plate, turning it over, and sliding it back into the pan, and let it cook on the other side for another 2 minutes without a lid. When the omelet has a denser consistency and a stronger color, turn off the heat, serve your shrimp omelet, and serve it hot or cold!

5) Potato pie in a pan

Ingredients:
- **Potatoes (about 1) 180 g**
- **Parmesan to grate 40 g**
- **Zucchini flowers 6**
- **Mozzarella 100 g**
- **Raw ham 100 g**

First, wash and dry the potatoes in their skins, slice them thinly and store them in a bowl full of water to prevent them from turning black. Take the zucchini flowers and cut off the stem, and detach the leaves from the flower base. To remove any earth residues inside the flower, gently wipe with a brush. Open the flower and remove the pistil. Cut the mozzarella into cubes and set aside. Now drain the potato slices and dry them with a cloth, heat a non-stick pan and arrange the first layer of potatoes on the spiral bottom, lay the potatoes overlapping them once you have made a circle, place a potato in the center so that there are no empty spaces between the slices. Sprinkle the whole surface with some of the cheese. Cover with the lid and heat for about 2-3 minutes. Spread another layer of potatoes in a spiral as you did previously, continue with a layer of cheese to cover the entire surface. Now stuff with half of the sliced ham, half of the zucchini flowers, and even half a dose of mozzarella cubes.

Continue with the remaining raw ham and the remaining zucchini flowers covered with the remaining mozzarella cubes and more cheese. Cover with the lid and let everything cook for about 10 minutes. Serve the potato pie in the pan immediately, so you can still enjoy it racy!

6) Saffron risotto

Ingredients:
- **Saffron in pistils 1 tsp**
- **Rice 320 g**
- **Vegetable butter 125 g**
- **Parmesan cheese to be grated 80 g**
- **Water q.s.**
- **Vegetable broth 1 l**
- **Salt up to taste**

First, put the saffron pistils in a small glass, pour enough water over the pistils to completely cover the pistils, mix and leave to infuse overnight; in this way, the pistils will release all their color. Then prepare the vegetable broth; for the recipe, you will need a liter. In a large pan, pour 50g of butter taken from the total dose required, melt it over low heat, then pour the rice and toast it for 3-4 minutes, so the grains will seal and keep cooking well. Next, proceed with cooking for about 18-20 minutes, adding the broth a ladle at a time, as needed, as the rice absorbs it: the grains must always be covered. Five minutes before the end of cooking, pour the water with the saffron pistils that you had infused, stir. Once cooked, turn off the heat, add salt, stir in the grated cheese and the remaining 75 g of butter, mix and cover with the lid on, let it rest for a couple of minutes. At this point, the saffron risotto is ready; serve it hot.

7) Cream of cauliflower

Ingredients:
- **Cauliflower 740 g**
- **Potatoes and 740 g**
- **Salt up to taste**
- **Extra virgin olive oil 3 tbsp**
- **Chives stem 1**
- **Vegetable butter 30 g**
- **Leeks 110 g**
- **Water 1 l**

Wash, peel and cut the potatoes into chunks, remove the green part of the leek and slice the white part into thin slices. Wash and clean the cauliflower; cut, with the help of a knife, the lower end of the head and remove the most rigid leaves, then remove the florets from the stem. Melt the butter with two tablespoons of oil in a saucepan. Add the leek, the cauliflower, the potatoes, and a liter of water and cook over medium heat for 10 minutes, occasionally stirring, then cover with a lid and continue cooking for another 20 minutes, over low heat. Once the vegetables are cooked, blend everything with the mixer. Chop the chives, sprinkle them on the cream, season with salt, and mix all the ingredients well. The cauliflower cream is ready: serve it hot, possibly accompanied by croutons of toasted bread, a drizzle of extra virgin olive oil, and grated Parmesan cheese.

8) Risotto with apples and speck

Ingredients:
- Rice 320 g
- Apples 2
- Raw ham 120 g (sliced)
- Vegetable broth to taste
- Vegetable butter 50 g
- Parmesan 50 g
- Rosemary to taste

First, prepare the vegetable broth and keep it warm. Then take the slices of ham and coarsely chopped. At this point, move on to the apples, cut them into 4 first, then peel them and cut them into cubes. To prevent them from blackening, dip them gradually in acidulated water. Pour half the butter dose into a pan, and the other will be used to whisk the risotto later. Melt the butter, then pour the rice inside. Toast it for a few minutes, always stirring. Begin to wet the rice with the hot broth and continue to do so only when needed. In another hot pan, pour a little oil, add both the ham and the apples, and sauté them over high heat. When the risotto is left to cook for about 3 minutes, pour apples and ham inside. As soon as the rice is cooked, turn off the heat and add the remaining butter and the Parmesan, sprinkling it all over the surface. Cover with a lid, wait 1 minute, stir gently, and shake the pan to finish stirring. Your risotto is ready, garnish with a few needles of rosemary and serve.

9) Cream of peas

Ingredients:
- **Peas 1 kg**
- **Fresh liquid cream 20 g**
- **Grated cheese 50 g**
- **Extra virgin olive oil 30 g**
- **Salt up to taste**
- **Vegetable broth 400 g**

In a pan, heat the oil over low heat, then add the peas, salt, and mix everything. Cook for about 5 minutes, then cover with 350 g of vegetable broth. Continue cooking for another 15-20 minutes, then turn off the heat and using an immersion blender, blend everything by adding the vegetable broth kept aside until it reaches a smooth consistency. Add the fresh cream, turn the heat back on and continue cooking for another 5 minutes, stirring often. Transfer your pea cream into a colander and sift it with the help of a spatula to make it even more creamy.

Serve your pea soup and garnish with Parmesan to taste before serving it hot or lukewarm as you prefer!

10) Pasta With Swordfish

Ingredients:
- **Spaghetti 320 g**
- **Olives 70 g**
- **Swordfish 300 g**
- **Cherry tomatoes 250 g**
- **Extra virgin olive oil 40 g**
- **Salt up to taste**

Start washing the tomatoes, then cut them into 4 parts and keep them aside. Take the swordfish steak, remove the skin using a sharp blade knife, and divide the steak in half if it is too thick. At this point, first, cut it into strips, and then these cut into cubes of about 1 cm each. Place a pan full of water, salted to taste, on the fire and bring it to the boil, and it will be used for cooking the pasta. Pour the olive oil into a pan, add the tomatoes, add salt, and let the tomatoes fry for a couple of minutes; then add a ladle of water (now hot), which will be used for cooking the pasta, and add the pitted olives. If the bottom dries out too much, add another ladle of cooking water and cook for another 2 minutes. In the meantime, throw the spaghetti into the boiling water, and while the pasta is cooking, add the swordfish cubes to the sauce, mix everything and cook for 5 minutes, adding another ladle of the cooking water. Drain the pasta directly in the sauce and toss it together with the sauce before serving!

11) Pasta with broccoli pesto

Ingredients:
- **Short pasta 320 g**
- **Coarse salt to taste**

FOR THE BROCCOLI PESTO
- **Broccoli 320 g**
- **Pine nuts 30 g**
- **Parmesan (for grating) 30 g**
- **Basil 10 g**
- **Extra virgin olive oil 70 g**
- **Salt up to 1 pinch**

Wash the broccoli, divide the florets from the central stem and let them blanch for 5 minutes, then drain and pour them into a bowl filled with water and ice to let them cool and keep the color alive. When the broccoli has cooled, drain it from the ice water and dry it with a paper towel. Transfer the broccoli to the mixer, add the basil leaves, pine nuts, grated Parmesan, a pinch of salt, and half of the extra virgin olive oil. Operate the blades to blend all the ingredients and add the remaining oil; if the mixture is too dry, add more oil. The pesto should be creamy; place it in a small bowl cover it with plastic wrap. Cook the pasta in plenty of boiling salted water.

Meanwhile, put the pesto in a large pan and dilute it with a ladle of the cooking water to softer. Drain the pasta and transfer it to the pan with the pesto. Let it cook over low heat for a few minutes, stirring with a spoon. The broccoli pesto pasta is ready to be brought to the table. Enjoy it now!

12) Mediterranean-style pasta salad

Ingredients:
- Short pasta 320 g
- Fresh basil 20 leaves
- Pitted black olives 40 g
- Natural tuna fillets (in jar) 200 g
- Mozzarella 200 g
- Corn in a jar
- Salt 1 pinch
- Extra virgin olive oil as needed

Cut the pitted olives into rounds and the mozzarella into cubes, which you will put in a colander to remove the excess whey. Meanwhile, bring a pot of salted water to a boil and throw in the pasta. In a large bowl, place the tuna and, with the tines of a fork, mash it to reduce it into strips. Add the hand-chopped basil leaves to the bowl with the tuna. Mix well to blend all the flavors. Drain the pasta and transfer it directly into the bowl together with the sauce. Also, add the black olives and mozzarella, which will have lost the excess liquid. If you prefer, mix well, season with a drizzle of extra virgin olive oil and a pinch of salt. Let your Mediterranean pasta salad rest for at least half an hour before bringing it to the table!

Chapter 9: Dessert

1) Baked Pears

Ingredients:
- **Pears 2**
- **Ricotta 200 g**
- **Spreadable cheese 80g**
- **Honey 40 g**
- **Chopped chives to taste**
- **Extra virgin olive oil as needed**
- **Salt up to taste**
- **Baked Pears**

First, wash and dry the fruits. Cut the pears in half for the long part and remove the core and a small part of the pulp. Remove a small part from the peel's side to be able to lay them more comfortably on the pan. Then place them on a baking sheet lined with parchment paper and season with a drizzle of oil and salt. Bake in a preheated static oven at 180 ° for 10 minutes or until they are sufficiently soft. Once cooked, remove from the oven and let it cool. Prepare the filling: pour the cream cheese, ricotta, salt into a bowl and blend with an immersion mixer until a smooth cream is obtained. Add the chopped chives, honey and mix with a spoon to emulsify. Stuff the cooked pears with the cream. Serve your baked pears immediately with gorgonzola and honey.

2) Apple Pie

Ingredients:
- **Apples 700 g**
- **Brown sugar 200 g**
- **00 flour 250 g**
- **Vegetable butter 100 g**
- **Skimmed milk (at room temperature) 150 g**
- **Eggs (at room temperature) 2**
- **Salt up to 1 pinch**
- **Baking powder**
- **Lemon 1**

Melt the butter in the microwave or a double boiler, and set aside. Peel the apples, cut them into slices and pour them into a bowl, and sprinkle them with the lemon juice, mixing them well: this will prevent them from blackening. Then sift the 00 flour with the baking powder. Then, in a large bowl, pour the eggs and part of the sugar dose. Start beating with the electric whisk and continue pouring the sugar a little at a time. When the mixture begins to lighten, add a pinch of salt and whip until the mixture is light and fluffy. At this point, add the melted butter brought back to room temperature. Then, continuing to whisk, add the sifted flour and baking powder one tablespoon at a time. When the powders are entirely incorporated, lower the electric whisk's speed and pour the milk slowly at room temperature. When the milk is completely incorporated, stop the whips: the dough is ready. Separately, drain the apples in a colander to remove the lemon juice and pour them into the mixture. Gently mix from bottom to top to incorporate them well. Grease and sprinkle with sugar a 22 cm diameter cake pan and pour the mixture. The cake is ready to be baked: bake it in a preheated static oven at 180 ° for about 55 minutes. When cooked, take it out of the oven and let it cool completely before removing it from the pan. Your apple pie is ready to be enjoyed!

3) Light cheesecake

Ingredients:
- **Wholemeal dry biscuits 180 g**
- **Light butter 80 g**

FOR THE CREAM
- **Light spreadable fresh cheese 500 g**
- **Low-fat yogurt 250 g**
- **Fructose 160 g**
- **Gelatin in sheets 10 g**
- **Water 30 g**
- **Vanilla bean 1**

Put the wholemeal biscuits in the mixer, then chop them finely. Place the shredded biscuits in a bowl. Now put the butter to melt in a saucepan; Gradually add the melted butter to the bowl in which you placed the chopped biscuits, mixing everything well until you get a sandy mixture. Butter a cake pan with a diameter of 24 cm; cut out a disc of parchment paper of the same diameter as the bottom of the pan and two strips of the same height as the edges, then lined. Pour the crumbled biscuits into the baking tray covered with parchment paper, and with the help of a spoon, compact the biscuit base well. Let the mixture cool in the refrigerator for half an hour or in the freezer for about ten minutes.

Now dedicate yourself to the filling: soften the gelatin sheets in cold water for about 10 minutes, squeeze them well. Meanwhile, place the spreadable cheese in a blender, add the fructose and operate the whisk to mix the ingredients. Then add the seeds of the vanilla bean. Incorporate the low-fat yogurt into the mixture and continue to mix with whips. In the meantime, the gelatine sheets will have softened well. Dissolve it in a saucepan with 30 g of hot water and when it has completely melted, incorporate it into the mixture of cheese and yogurt. Mix all the ingredients well with the hand whisk to obtain a homogeneous and creamy mixture. At this point, the cream is ready; pour it on the biscuit base, now cold and compact. Smooth out the cream to level it out. Then put your light cheesecake in the refrigerator for at least 4 hours to make it firm, and then serve it!

4) Coconut biscuits

Ingredients:
- **Rapè coconut 150 g**
- **Brown sugar 120 g**
- **Egg whites 3**

Pour the rapé coconut into a bowl, add the sugar, mix and add the egg whites. Mix everything thoroughly: you will have to work until you get a uniform mixture. Then take small parts of the dough with a spoon and transfer them to a drip pan already lined with parchment paper. Make about 18 cookies. Bake in a preheated convection oven at 200 ° for about 10 minutes or until they are golden on the surface. Take them out of the oven and let them cool. Once cold, serve your coconut sweets!

5) Carrot treats

Ingredients:
- **Carrots 250 g**
- **Brown sugar 200 g**
- **00 flour 250 g**
- **Potato starch 50 g**
- **Eggs 1**
- **Yolks 1**
- **Seed oil 130 ml**
- **Orange peel 1**
- **Vanilla bean 1**
- **Powdered yeast 8 g**

Start by washing the carrots well and peeling them, then chop them finely in a blender. In a large bowl, whip the eggs with the sugar. When the mixture is light and fluffy, add the chopped carrots. Sift the flour, potato starch, yeast and add them to the egg and sugar mixture. Finally, add the zest of an orange and the seeds of a vanilla bean. Then add the seed oil to the mixture, mixing well; the dough must be very soft. Line 12 muffin molds (diameter of about 6/7 cm) with paper cups (or butter and flour them) and pour the carrot mixture into each mold, leaving about a centimeter from the top. Bake the patties in a preheated static oven at 180 ° C for about 20/25 minutes, until inserting a stick in the center of one of the patties and extracting it; it will not be dry.

Cool, remove them from the molds, and serve.

6) Water cake

Ingredients:
- **Natural water, at room temperature 330 g**
- **00 flour 300 g**
- **Brown sugar 200 g**
- **Powdered yeast 16 g**
- **Seed oil 90 g**
- **Vanilla bean 1**

Start by sifting the flour with the yeast into a bowl and set aside for a moment. In another bowl, pour the sugar and add the water at room temperature, stirring well with a whisk to dissolve the sugar. With a knife, cut a vanilla pod lengthwise and collect the seeds, which you will add to the water and sugar. At this point, add the seed oil and mix. Now take the sifted powders and add them, a spoon at a time, to the emulsion of water, sugar, and oil, always mixing well and continuously to avoid the creation of lumps. Once you have added all the flour, you will get a soft, smooth, and lump-free dough. Take a 24 cm diameter mold and line it with baking paper. Or, if you prefer, you can simply oil and flour it with a little seed oil and a tablespoon of flour. When the mold is ready, pour the cake mixture into it.

Bake in a preheated static oven at 180 ° for 50 minutes. If cooking seems to you that the cake is too colored, after the first half hour of cooking, cover the cake with a sheet of aluminum foil and continue cooking. Before taking out the oven, test the toothpick: if it comes out clean and dry, it means that the cake is cooked correctly. Remove the cake and let it cool. Your water cake is ready to be enjoyed!

7) Soft ricotta and pear cake

Ingredients:
- Pears 400 g
- Cow's milk ricotta 350 g
- 00 flour 250 g
- Powdered yeast for cakes 16 g
- Eggs 3
- Brown sugar 170 g
- Lemon zest 1
- Vanilla bean 1

Cut the pears into instead small cubes, put them in a bowl with very little lemon juice to prevent them from blackening. Beat the sugar with the ricotta with a whisk (or in a planetary mixer), then add the vanilla pod's seeds. Then incorporate the 3 eggs one by one and continue to whip the mixture; add the grated lemon zest. Sift the flour with the baking powder and add them to the mixture, mixing with a wooden spoon until you get a smooth dough. Incorporate the diced pears and mix them with the dough. Grease and flour a pan with a diameter of 24 cm well, pour in the cake dough, and level it well with the help of a spatula. At this point, bake the cake at 180 ° C for 50/70 minutes, until by introducing a wooden toothpick in the center of the cake, it will be dry. If the cake gets too dark on the surface during cooking, cover it with aluminum foil. Take the soft ricotta and pear cake out of the oven, let it cool, turn it out of the mold and sprinkle it and serve!

8) Honey cake

Ingredients:
- **Honey 250 g**
- **00 flour 200 g**
- **White yogurt 110 g**
- **Vegetable butter 65 g**
- **Potato starch 50 g**
- **Eggs 3**
- **Powdered yeast for cakes 16 g**
- **Orange peel 1**

Lightly heat the honey in a saucepan, remove from the heat and add the butter and yogurt. Separately separate the egg whites from the yolks and add the latter to the honey mixture. Mix with a whisk until you obtain a homogeneous mixture that you will transfer to a bowl. Now sift the flour, starch, cinnamon, and baking powder separately. Add the powders to the honey mixture, mix it, season with the grated orange peel, and set aside.

Preheat the oven to 200 ° in static mode, then take the egg whites kept aside and whisk them with an electric whisk until they are frothy, at which point add the mixture to the whipped egg whites and mix gently with the spatula from the bottom up. High until a homogeneous mixture is obtained. Grease and flour a 22 cm diameter mold and fill it with the dough. Now you can bake the honey cake in a preheated static oven at 200 ° for 40 minutes. When cooked, take your cake out of the oven, let it cool, then turn it out and serve.

9) Sweet zucchini pie

Ingredients:
- Zucchini 300 g
- 00 flour 350 g
- Eggs 3
- Corn oil 200 ml
- Brown sugar 250 g
- Baking powder for cakes 1 sachet
- Vanilla bean 1

Start by washing the zucchini, removing the ends, and grating them. Beat the whole eggs with the sugar until the mixture is light and fluffy; add the flour and the well sifted yeast. Then, they also beat the seeds of the vanilla pod. Also, add the seed oil, mixing well to mix it, and finally the grated zucchini. Mix everything and pour the mixture into a buttered and floured pan of 24/26 cm (or covered with parchment paper). Bake the zucchini cake for about 60 minutes at 180 ° C. If the surface becomes too dark after the first 40 minutes of cooking, cover it with aluminum foil. Let the zucchini sweet cake cool before turning it out.

10) Peach cake

Ingredients:
- **Peaches (cleaned 285 g) 330 g**
- **00 flour 280 g**
- **Brown sugar 170 g**
- **Seed oil 90 g**
- **Skimmed milk at room temperature 90 g**
- **3 eggs at room temperature 155 g**
- **Powdered yeast for cakes 16 g**
- **Lemon zest 1**

Start by lighting the oven at 180 °, then wash the peaches under running water, dry them, and cut them into reasonably coarse pieces: you will need 285 g of peach pulp. Carefully weigh all the ingredients and pour them into the mixer: first, pour the peaches into wedges, sugar, flour, whole eggs, yeast, flavored with lemon zest, and finally pour in the liquids: seed oil and milk. Operate the blades and blend everything until you get a creamy mixture. Grease and flour a 22 cm diameter cake pan and pour the mixture inside. The dough is ready for cooking. Bake in a preheated oven at 180 degrees for 60 minutes. When cooked, take the peach pan out of the oven and cool it before cutting it into slices.

11) Yogurt smoothie

Ingredients:
- **Low-fat yogurt 250 g**
- **Lime juice (about 1) 13 g**
- **Pulp melon 420**
- **Peaches pulp 350 g**

First, wash the peaches (it will take about 3), peel and remove the stone, cut them into coarse pieces, and set them aside to prepare the yogurt smoothie. Now take care of the melon: cut it in half, remove the seeds and peel, then cut it into pieces. Cut the lime in half and squeeze it with the help of a juicer. Collect the juice obtained in a glass and keep it aside. Now take a blender and place the melon and peaches. Pour in the yogurt and lime juice, close the blender and turn it on. Continue to blend until you get a creamy mixture. Your freshest yogurt smoothie is ready!

12) Baked apples

Ingredients:
- Apples 4
- Brown sugar 40 g
- Honey 1 tbsp
- Ground cinnamon 1 tsp
- Sugar 1 tsp
- Lemons 1
- Water 50 g

To make baked apples, first cut the lemon into wedges and set it aside. Remove the peel from the apples, remove the core and internal seeds, then remove any residual peel with a small knife. Pass on the peeled apples' surface a lemon wedge so that they do not blacken. Pour the brown sugar into a bowl and roll the apples here so that the sugar sticks all over the surface. Place the apples on an ovenproof dish that contains them well. Sprinkle the remaining brown sugar on the surface, making it also penetrate the apple's inner part. Spread the cinnamon through a sieve and pour the water into the pan's bottom to prevent the apples from sticking or the sugar from burning. Bake the apples in the preheated static oven at 200 ° C for 30 minutes. After the indicated cooking time, remove the pan and pour 1 tablespoon of honey onto the apples' surface to make them even shinier.

Bake again for another 10 minutes, again at 200 ° C. When cooked, take the pan with the baked apples out of the oven and sprinkle with sugar to make them even more inviting. Serve the baked apples while still hot, drizzled with the cooking juices.

Conclusion

Gastritis is used to describe a group of disorders with one feature in common, inflammation of the gastric mucosa. Today, in fact, in addition to being a discomfort that affects men and women of every race, age, and social rank, gastritis manifests itself in different forms: some gastritis sufferers complain of simple and temporary heartburn; in others, however, the disorder causes aerophagia, dyspepsia, loss of appetite, up to degenerate into severe and disabling symptoms such as diarrhea, abdominal cramps, meteorism, halitosis, and vomiting. The triggering cause intensely conditions the type of symptoms and the intensity with which they occur. Fortunately, in most cases, mild gastritis is quickly resolved with lifestyle correction. Other times, however, where the disease takes on a chronic or particularly aggressive connotation, the therapy must be more drastic. In both cases, especially if intense, the malaise felt must not be neglected but submitted to the attention of the doctor, both to avoid unnecessary suffering and because, even in a minority of people, the onset of heartburn, cramps, and Abdominal pain can be a sign of a more severe condition that can pose significant risks to overall health. It is advisable to change your lifestyle and diet, and this guide offers many useful tips on preventing gastritis with proper nutrition.

GERD Diet Cookbook
Introduction
GERD also called gastric reflux or stomach acid and is a digestive system disorder. It can damage the esophagus, and heartburn is the main symptom of this condition. The esophagus is used for swallowing, and the disease occurs when the acid contained in the stomach returns through the esophagus and inflames it. If you have acid reflux, you may develop a sour or bitter taste in the mouth, and it may cause you to regurgitate food or liquid from the stomach.

One of the causes of GERD is poor nutrition, little variety of diet, little physical activity, lack of sleep, and stress. The best way to treat GERD symptoms is a radical change in lifestyle without smoking and alcohol. Follow a diet and exercise; they can help overcome acid reflux and improve their digestive health.

Studies have shown that between 21 and 40% of people suffer from heartburn. More than 60 million adult Americans suffer from heartburn at least once a month. Although acid reflux occurs in both women and men, men have been shown to have more GERD symptoms. This book will provide you with many helpful tips on GERD, causes, symptoms, and numerous recipes for getting back to eating without pleasure. That annoying post-meal heartburn. In addition to a healthy diet, we will give particular attention to the correct lifestyle made of sports activities, the importance of sleeping, and reducing stress.

Chapter 1: Gastro-Esophageal Reflux Disease

Gastroesophageal reflux disease is often caused by reflux into the esophagus of stomach contents and intestinal gases that generate gastroesophageal reflux. This leads to heartburn or throat burning. Occasional small refluxes are considered physiological, for example, once a week, but if the symptom is repeated several times during the week, medical assistance must be requested.

Causes

GERD is caused due to multiple factors. GERD is caused by numerous factors. It is important to know and identify these reasons and problems. When you are aware of the causes, it is easier to change your lifestyle and improve yourself.
Here are the main causes of GERD:

Obesity

Obesity is a clinical condition in which the subject has significant accumulations of body fat. This can compromise vital functions and lead to a deterioration in the quality of life. Weight gain can cause problems with bones, body resistance, heart performance, blood circulation, and organ activities. The obese person has an increased abdominal circumference and therefore, an elevated abdominal pressure, which favors the ascent of gastric juices into the esophagus and promotes sphincter incontinence.

Alcohol
Alcohol is another important cause of GERD. Alcohol is, in fact, already dangerous in itself on people's health. It has been observed that high consumption of alcoholic beverages not only causes acid reflux but increases the risk of a pre-cancerous lesion of the esophagus and the tumor itself.

Smoke
Smoking is one of the biggest causes of GERD. Smoking affects not only the lungs but also the stomach because nicotine stimulates acid secretion. The combined effect of caffeine and nicotine causes an even higher increase in gastric acidity.

Low physical activity
As mentioned before, overweight and the consequent increase in the abdominal part is a cause of GERD, so a little physical activity during the week is good for you. You train correctly, with a specific program to your fitness, also following a specific nutritional plan. A healthy diet associated with exercise will be your allies in alleviating symptoms and reducing the probability of complications; your overall health will improve, and your quality of life will definitely have a positive turnaround.

Diet does not vary
Poor variety in the diet can have a negative effect on your overall health, and GERD can be caused by poor food options. If you consume junk food, snacks, soft drinks, high-fat foods, you may experience acid reflux.

Bad habits and incorrect posture
GERD can also occur from bad habits such as incorrect posture while eating, such as eating while lying down. Another bad habit is to go to lie on a bed or on the sofa after each meal. It is advisable to take a short walk after eating or at least not to go to bed immediately.

Pregnancy
GERD is one of the most common ailments in pregnancy because of hormonal changes and the position of the fetus. Usually, this is a problem that mostly affects the past three months.

Medications
Medications can lead to GERD as a side effect, including nonsteroidal anti-inflammatory drugs, aspirin, and some antibiotics.

Symptoms
Being aware of the symptoms is essential for healthy living, and starting to understand that we are suffering from GERD. As soon as we feel the symptoms of acid reflux, we must immediately act accordingly to avoid even serious complications. Here are a few major symptoms of gastric acid reflux to consider:

-Heartburn is the most common symptom. It appears as a burning sensation under the chest bone. Pain is caused by irritation of the lining of the esophagus due to the passage of acid that has risen from the stomach.

-Bitter in the back of the mouth and throat

-Burning throat in the upper part

-Even bloody and painful nausea and vomiting in severe cases

-GERD can cause very dark and bleeding stools, accompanied by burning

-Prolonged hiccups accompanied by burning and pain in the throat.

-Feeling that food is stuck in the throat.

-Difficulty in swallowing food, with pain and burning

-Sore throat, a dry cough can occur in the early stages.

-Halitosis and dental erosion are other main symptoms of GERD.

GERD can begin to present itself from the simple burp to the bloody vomit; therefore, one should not take to read these symptoms listed above, even the banalest. It is essential to identify these symptoms initially and to take immediate measures to quickly resolve these problems. Each of the above symptoms does not necessarily address all of them at once, but the symptoms are likely to occur from time to time. So it is important to pay attention to the initial symptoms as well.

Sometimes you may have these problems along with other medical conditions, so be sure to discuss them with your doctor first.

Treatments

GERD is one of the most common digestive disorders involving millions of people around the world. When gastric reflux is not treated properly, it can produce hiatal hernia. It prevents the functioning of the diaphragm regulating valve, which has the task of controlling the flow of food and keeping food in the stomach. You should not underestimate the symptoms in order not to have complications later in your life. It is necessary to chase after treatments. As soon as possible.

Here is some treatment option:

Lifestyle
Sometimes simply changing your lifestyle is enough to get better in many health conditions. Specifically for GERD, you have to avoid some habits that many people in the world have, including:
stop smoking
abuse of alcohol
Eat quickly by chewing a little
follow a light diet with few or no spices
eat small meals and at intervals of time
lose weight
avoid chewing gum
bedtime
Dress in tight clothes
Perform substantial physical efforts immediately after meals
avoid bedtime immediately after eating

Natural treatments

There are some natural remedies for Gerd that include easily available supplements and herbs. However, they may be useful in combination with what your doctor recommends for GERD

Below is a list of herbs and supplements:

- Ginger root

    is one of the most common natural supplements for stomach problems. It relaxes the muscles in the esophagus and calms the digestive tract. Ginger also improves digestion and consequently helps reduce GERD or reflux because food and acid do not persist in the stomach.

- Licorice root
    calms the stomach. It reduces inflammation of the lining of the esophagus and stomach, which is caused by GERD. It stimulates the body's natural defense mechanisms and is a natural anti-inflammatory.

- Lavender
    its antispasmodic properties it is known to promote proper digestion and to limit the presence of gas in the gastrointestinal level. It is mainly used as an infusion.

- Chicory
    the root can be a very useful digestive aid for people who have GERD. Chicory is also effective

for relieving reflux pain because it helps relax the stomach.

- Antioxidants
  antioxidant vitamins A, C, and E are recognized for their potential in preventing GERD. Vitamin supplements are usually used if not enough nutrients are received from food. A blood test can help determine which nutrients your body needs. Your doctor may also prescribe a multivitamin.

- Melatonin
  as the "sleep hormone," melatonin is a hormone produced in the pineal gland. This gland is located in the brain. Melatonin is primarily known for helping initiate sleep.

- Aloe vera
  in reducing the main reflux symptoms

Medications
- In the early stages of GERD, there are some medications you can use, so remember that you need to consult your doctor before undertaking any drug treatments. With medications, the

  aim is to reduce esophageal acidity, neutralizing the acid produced, or inhibiting its upstream production. There are different types of medications for gastroesophageal reflux (antacids, histaminergic receptor blockers, proton pump inhibitors) If not in serious cases, it is always to avoid taking them before using them and triggering the vicious circle. It would be good to consider other ways: diet, lifestyle, exercise, reduction of stress, and cigarette smoking. Make sure to consult the physician in severe cases for the medication prescription and regular checkups.

Risks and complications

If you underestimate the problem and delay with treatments, you can chase complications and risks. Potential complications of GERD include:
- Esophageal stenosis, which occurs when the esophagus narrows or narrows
- Esophagitis (inflammation of the esophagus)
- Esophageal cancer, which affects a small portion of people with Barrett's esophagus
- Barrett's esophagus, which involves permanent changes to the lining of your esophagus
- Erosion of tooth enamel, gum disease.
- Asthma, chronic cough or other breathing problems

It is essential to solving the problem in the first phase to have adequate and easy-to-perform treatment, thus avoiding reaching more extreme solutions.

Chapter 2: Prevention from GERD

Yes, prevention is better than cure. You need to make sure you take some essential precautions that will help you live a healthy life. GERD is not caused by external factors such as viruses or infections but only by a wrong daily routine. With a little attention, it is quite easy to follow the prevention guide for GERD related problems.

Foods to eat and avoid

Most of the problems caused by GERD are related to poor nutrition, so it is necessary to follow a healthy and light diet. Eating correctly is the best method to prevent gastric reflux and allow you to have positive and tangible results in a short period. Now let's see how healthy food can become a valuable ally for prevention, and we will find out what foods to eat and avoid.

What not to eat

Avoid high-fat foods. These are difficult to digest, and this means they stay in the stomach longer. When foods slow down digestion, the chances of them returning to the esophagus increase, leading to reflux.

To avoid this situation, you need to avoid foods such as:
- Animal fat such as lard, bacon, hamburger, pork fat cuts, cold cuts, hot dog, etc
- High-fat snacks that do not have much nutritional value, such as chips, candy, or ice cream.
- Fried foods such as chips, vegetable fries and fried chicken
- salmon, octopus, cuttlefish, mussels, clams, etc.

Protein foods raw or overcooked come:

- Ragout or similar
- Carpaccio, tartare, sushi, etc.
- Braised

Eat less acidic foods:
- Tomato and juice
- Citrus fruits and juice.
- Vinegar

High-calorie foods that can promote overweight:
- Very seasoned foods
- Cheeses
- pasta in an abundant portion

Spices and flavorings
- Chili pepper
- Onion and garlic(In ample quantities)
- Pepper
- All carbonated drinks.

The techniques not recommended are:
- Brazing
- Frying in a pan
- Stewing

Foods to eat

The following are the foods that must be part of the diet daily to prevent GERD:
- Among the recommended meats there are: chicken, rabbit, turkey, defatted pork or beef muscle, etc
- Among the fishery products: cod, anchovies, sea bream, sea bass, tuna fillet, prawns, etc.
- Among the cheeses: lean ricotta, light spreadable cheese, cottage cheese.
- Among legumes, cereals and derivatives, choose those with medium or low fiber content.

- fruits and vegetables

The recommended cooking techniques are:
- Steam-powered
- In a pressure cooker
- Boil in water
- Baked
- Grilled
- In a pan over low heat.

By following these dietary guidelines, you will take a big step forward to prevent GERD and have a healthy life.

Impact of Exercise

In the prevention of GERD, physical activity has a significant impact; as it is done after 2/3 hours after the main meal, it will consume all or part of the energy consumed by the food. It will also help you have faster digestion and consequently avoid acid reflux.

Weight reduction

Overweight or obesity are some of the reasons that can lead to GERD. Regular physical activity will lead to a decrease in weight associated with the correct diet. In general, reducing weight will help you have a better quality of life.

An active mind and healthy body

An excellent physical activity routine is an excellent combination of body and mind. With daily training, you will consume a lot of your strength and release a lot of the tension you have. With the effort due to a workout, our brain will release the stress hormone, and this will make for a good night's sleep.

Activate the repair muscles
Exercise and exertion activate the repairing muscles in the body, which help reduce internal and external inflammation. Exercise helps manage this painful condition and enables the body to repair damaged cells.

Lifestyle changes
To prevent GERD, it is necessary to make changes to your lifestyle, as mentioned in the previous pages. These changes not only help prevent the acid reflux problem but will also give you a better life and avoid further health problems.

Eat healthily
Healthy eating is the top priority. If you eat fatty foods, refined sugars must be replaced immediately. These foods must be consumed very rarely, only in rare situations. It is necessary to introduce healthy and light food among your food options to avoid such problems.

Plan your meals
Organizing your meals is essential for the prevention of GERD. Waiting too much between meals is never healthy because it leads to massive meals and consequently, prolonged digestion. It is advisable to make small meals, eat little, and often with meals scheduled with specific intervals that reduce the risk of GERD.

Do not sleep immediately after a meal
Going to sleep shortly after eating is a bad habit that must be eliminated. The possibility of acid reflux increases as the position taken when sleeping does not guarantee proper digestion.

Maintain a balance between food options
Changing lifestyles does not mean abandoning all food options. Some foods should be favored over others, but the important thing is knowing how to balance food options and not just eating the same things all the time. Make sure you have many choices in your diet. That will help you have the right food balance.

Sleep well
Sleep is essential for digestion and stomach food to function well. Sleep is vital to allow digested food and stomach to work well. Make sure you sleep well at least between 7/8 hours. Sleeping little will make you feel tired and will not encourage you to want to exercise.

Do not stress yourself
Stress and anxiety can affect the proper functioning of the digestive system. Anxiety and stress have effects that fall on the stomach. A stressed brain negatively affects the general function of the organism.

Chapter 3: Recipes for breakfast

1) Maple syrup pancakes

Ingredients:
- Butter vegetable 25 g
- 00 flour 125 g
- Medium eggs 2
- Fresh whole milk 200 g
- Baking powder for cakes 6 g
- Brown sugar 15 g

TO SEAL:
Maple syrup to taste

We begin the preparation of pancakes by melting the butter on shallow heat, then let it cool. Meanwhile, divide the egg whites from the yolks. Pour the yolks into a bowl and beat them with a hand whisk, then add the melted butter at room temperature and the milk flush, continuing to mix with the whisk. Whisk the mixture until it becomes clear. Add the yeast to the flour and sift everything in the bowl with the egg mixture, mix with the whisk to blend. Now whip the egg whites that you have kept aside, pouring the sugar little by little, and when they are white and frothy, gently add them to the egg mixture, with movements from top to bottom, to avoid disassembling them. Heat over medium heat (not high; otherwise you will not give the dough time to rise well during cooking, and the pancakes will become too dark) a large non-stick pan (preferably with a thick bottom) and, if necessary, grease with a little butter to spread on the surface with the help of kitchen paper. Pour a ladle of preparation into the center of the saucepan; there will be no need to spread it. When bubbles begin to appear on the surface, and the base will be golden, turn it on the other side using a spatula, as if it were a crepe or an omelet, then brown the other side in turn, after which the pancake will be ready. Continue with the rest of the dough, and gradually arrange the pancakes on a serving plate, stack them one on top of the other. About 12 pancakes should form with these doses. Serve them hot and sprinkled with maple syrup. You can accompany the pancakes with fresh fruit or sugar of your taste.

2) Muffin with chocolate drops

Ingredients:

- **Vegetable butter at room temperature 125 g**
- **almond flour 265 g**
- **135 g brown sugar**
- **Skimmed milk at room temperature 135 g**
- **Eggs (about 2) at room temperature 110 g**
- **Dark chocolate drops 100 g**
- **Vanilla bean 1**
- **1 tsp frosted bicarbonate**
- **Add a pinch of salt**
- **Baking powder 1**

To prepare the muffins with chocolate chips worked with the electric whisk butter, left to soften at room temperature for at least an hour previously, with the sugar, until obtaining a frothy and creamy mixture. Then cut a vanilla bean and scrape the seeds using the back of a knife. Pour the latter into the bowl with butter and sugar. Operate the whips again and add the eggs, also at room temperature, one at a time in this way the ingredients will not untie. Now sift the flour, baking powder, and baking soda directly into the bowl with the mixture. Also, add a pinch of salt and operate the whisk again to incorporate the powders. You will notice that the dough will become more consistent, then dilute it with milk at room temperature poured flush. At this point, the mixture will be soft and compact. Add 80 grams of chocolate chips and mix them with a spatula to incorporate them.

Then transfer the mixture into a disposable bag without nozzle; in this way, you can do a cleaner job; otherwise, use a spoon as well. Place the paper cups in a muffin pan and fill them 2/3 full, leaving less than an inch from the surface. Each muffin will have to weigh approximately 70 grams. Pour the remaining 20 drops of chocolate over the cupcakes and bake in a preheated oven at 180 ° for 18-20 minutes in static mode (otherwise at 160 ° for 13-15 minutes if the oven is ventilated). At this point, your chocolate chip muffins are ready to be enjoyed.

3) Yoghurt plum cake

Ingredients:
- 00 flour 300 g
- Eggs (about 5) 300 g
- Light butter 200 g
- 200 g powdered sugar
- Low-fat yogurt 150 g
- Potato starch 50 g
- Powdered yeast for cakes 15 g
- Vanilla bean seeds 1
- Salt up to 4 g

FOR MOLDS
- Butter to taste
- 00 flour to taste

To prepare the yogurt plumcake, equip yourself with a mixer equipped with fairly powerful and capacious blades. Place the cubed butter, the seeds of the vanilla bean, the eggs and the flour in the container yogurt, icing sugar, salt, yeast, and starch. Work at maximum speed for about 4 minutes. In the meantime, grease and flour two 16x8 cm slightly flared molds. As soon as you have obtained a homogeneous mixture, transfer it into the molds. Now dip a blade of a knife, first in the melted butter and then in the center of the two plumcakes. This will ensure uniform growth in cooking. Now put the plumcake in a preheated static oven, and they will have to cook in 2 phases: first at 185 ° for 15 minutes, then at

165 ° for 30 minutes. As soon as they are cooked, take them out of the oven and let them cool completely. At this point, turn them out and decorate them with icing sugar, and your yogurt plumcakes are ready to taste.

4) Vegetable tart

Ingredients:

- 1 pack of puff pastry of about 300 g
- 2 zucchini
- 4 potatoes
- 4 eggs
- 30 g of grated cheese
- basil
- chives
- extra virgin olive oil
- salt

To make the vegetable tart, start cutting the zucchini. Cut the two ends of the zucchini and cut into slices of about 5mm thick. Salt them slightly and let them drain in a colander. Peel the potatoes, wash and dry them, then cut as if you should make some fried chips by transferring them to a pan in which you have heated two tablespoons of oil. Brown the potatoes and cook them for 10 minutes. Remove from the heat and put them on paper towels. In the same pan, place the well-dried zucchini and prepare it by turning it often for 15 minutes. In the meantime, beat the eggs. Cook the zucchini, put them in a bowl, add the potatoes and mix everything with the beaten eggs, the grated cheese, the basil, chopped and salted chives. Brush a tart pan with oil and lay the puff pastry on it. Distribute the filling prepared evenly and bake in a hot oven at 200 ° for about 25 minutes. Then leave the vegetable tart to rest for about ten minutes and serve.

5) Potato omelette

Ingredients:

- **Eggs 6**
- **Potatoes 500 g**
- **Parmesan cheese 100 g**
- **Parsley to taste**
- **Salt to taste**
- **Seed oil to taste**

To make the potato omelet, first, put some water in a pan and bring to the boil. In the meantime, peel the potatoes and slice them. Now boil the potatoes for about 5 minutes. When cooking the potatoes finely chopped parsley. Now pour the eggs into a bowl, the chopped parsley, the grated cheese, and then salt At this point, mix to mix the ingredients. Drain the potatoes that have finished cooking, let them cool, and then add them to the egg mixture. Now go to cooking: in a pan heat a drizzle of seed oil, and once it is hot, pour the mixture. Cover with the lid and cook over moderate heat for 15 minutes, turning the pan occasionally.

When the surface is not very soft but still damp, turn the omelet over the lid, rotating the pan upside down with a decisive and rapid movement. Slide the omelet back into the pan to cook the other side, cover again with the lid and continue cooking for another 5 minutes. After this time, the omelet will be ready. You can serve it hot or cold.

6) Apple heart biscuits

Ingredients:
- an egg
- 100 g of cane sugar
- half a bag of yeast
- wholemeal flour to taste
- a coffee glass of extra virgin olive oil
- grated orange peel

For the apple filling
- 3 apples
- 2 teaspoons of powdered ginger
- the juice of half a lemon
- 2 tablespoons of brown sugar

In a bowl, put the egg, brown sugar, grated orange peel, and olive oil. Mix the ingredients with a fork in a circular and continuous pattern until you get a homogeneous and creamy mixture. Stir in the yeast and mix. At this point, add the sifted flour a little at a time, always mixing it with a fork in the bowl. You will see the dough gradually transform, acquire body and shape while remaining soft. For the recipe's success, this is an important step: consider mixing the flour at the rate of a spoon at a time until your liquid and creamy dough become more compact but not hard. Transfer it to a lightly floured pastry board and knead. When it no longer sticks to your hands, your pastry will be ready. Give it a ball shape and place it in the refrigerator for 30 minutes.

7) Apple muffin

Ingredients:

- **Apples 310 g**
- **00 flour 300 g**
- **Greek yogurt 150 g**
- **Sugar 120 g**
- **Eggs (about 4) 220 g**
- **Baking powder for sweets 16 g**
- **Lemon zest 1**

Start by pouring the eggs into a large bowl and start whipping them with forks or with an electric whisk, then add the sugar little by little continuing to work for about 5 minutes. Add the yogurt and mix it again with the whisk. Sift the yeast and flour into a separate bowl and add them a spoon at a time, keeping the whisk in action. Finally, add the grated lemon zest and mix again. Now wash the apples, cut them into wedges, and remove the peel. Cut the wedges into cubes and add them to the dough, then mix with a spatula to incorporate them evenly. Line a muffin pan with paper cups and fill them with about two tablespoons of dough each. Bake in a preheated static oven at 180 ° for about 25-28 minutes. Once cooked, take it out of the oven and let it cool. Your apple muffins are ready to taste!

8) Baked Frittata

Ingredients:

- **Eggs 8**
- **Grated cheese 100 g**
- **Chives to taste**
- **Thyme to taste**
- **Salt to taste**
- **Extra virgin olive oil 10 g**

FOR BRUSHING AND SPREADING THE TRAY

- **Extra virgin olive oil to taste**
- **Breadcrumbs to taste**

To prepare the frittata, start by oiling a 26x19 cm rectangular baking dish, then line it with breadcrumbs 2. Beat the eggs, add the grated cheese, oil, finely chopped chives. Continue with peeled thyme, salt. Then keep on beating for a few moments until a homogeneous mixture is obtained. Transfer everything to the oven dish and cook in a preheated static oven at 170 ° for 25 minutes. Once ready, serve your frittata in the hot oven to start the day!

9) Porridge

Ingredients:

- **Oat flakes 140 g**
- **Skimmed milk 220 g220 g**
- **Water 200 g**
- **Salt to taste**

TO SEAL
- **Honey to taste**
- **Strawberries to taste**
- **Flaked almonds to taste**

To make the porridge first, pour the oats into a bowl, cover with water and leave to soak for about an hour, (it is preferable to leave it to soak the night before). Pour the oats into the saucepan, add the milk, add a pinch of salt and cook the mixture for about 4-5 minutes, stirring often. When the oats are soft and have absorbed the milk, turn off the heat and transfer the porridge to a bowl and flavor with the honey. Garnish with slices of fresh strawberries and almonds. Serve your lukewarm porridge.

10) Salted Plumcake

Ingredients:
- Corn flour 200 g
- Eggs 3
- Raw ham 150 g
- Skimmed milk 150 ml
- Extra virgin olive oil 60 ml
- Salt to taste
- Instant yeast for savory preparations 1 sachet
- Grated cheese 150 g

To prepare the salted plumcake, start by sifting the yeast and flour in a bowl, then add the grated cheese. Mix the ingredients well and stir in the raw ham, mix again. Then add the extra virgin olive oil flush. In another bowl, beat the eggs with the milk and salt and add the liquid, thus obtained to the mixture of flour, cheese, and ham. Stir with a spoon until the ingredients are well mixed. Grease and flour a plumcake mold with a capacity of one liter and put the dough inside. Level it with the back of a spoon and bake in a preheated oven at 180 ° C for 45/50 minutes, doing a toothpick test to check its cooking. When the salted plumcake is cooked, wait until it is warm before removing it from the mold, then let it cool completely. Serve your salted plumcake!

Chapter 4: Recipes for starter

1) Boiled eggs

Ingredients:

- **4 fresh eggs**

To prepare the hard-boiled eggs, start by placing the whole eggs in a large saucepan and pour the cold water (the water will have to cover the eggs). Then put the saucepan on the fire and let it boil. From the boil, calculate 9 minutes of cooking. After 9 minutes, remove the saucepan from the heat and pass it under fresh running water to cool the eggs. This will allow you to peel them without getting burned; carefully remove all the shells, then divide the eggs in half, and you will discover the perfectly cooked interior! Boiled eggs are ready to be eaten as you like!

2) Gratinated prawns

Ingredients:

- Gratinated prawns
- Shrimp (about 16) 200 g
- Salt to taste
- White wine 80 ml
  FOR THE PANURE
- Breadcrumbs 50 g
- Parmesan 25 g
- Extra virgin olive oil to taste
- Parsley to be chopped 10 g
- Salt to taste

We start cleaning the shellfish by peeling them and leaving the tail, cut the back of the shrimp with a knife to eliminate the black thread inside. Place two prawns in each shell (or in any container of your imagination), to occupy the interior, and pour a spoonful of white wine into each one, directly on the prawns. To prepare the panure: in a bowl, arrange the breadcrumbs, the chopped parsley, the grated Parmesan, and the salt. Pour a drizzle of oil and mix. Cover the shells with a few tablespoons of panure and add a drizzle of oil. Arrange the shells with the prawns on a baking tray covered with parchment paper and bake at 180 degrees for about 25 minutes. Now you are ready to serve this imaginative dish!

3) Pineapple stuffed with shrimp

Ingredients:

- **Pineapple of about 1 kg 1**
- **Shrimp 450 g**
- **Chives 6 strands**
- **Mint 5 leaves**
- **Extra virgin olive oil to taste**
- **Salt to taste**
- **Mixed salad**

Let's start by cleaning the shrimp (you can also use the frozen ones), eliminating the fillet inside. Rinse them under running water, then lift your head with your hands and lift your legs. At this point, shell them. Once all the prawns have been cleaned, pour a drizzle of oil into a large pan. Add the peeled shrimp to the pan and brown them on both sides. Then turn off the heat and put them in a small bowl to cool them. Prepare the pineapple that will be the salad's container: choose a ripe pineapple and divide it in half. Cut the inner pulp along the perimeter of both halves to extract all the pulp without breaking it. Eliminate the most callused part of the pulp. From the extracted pulp, obtain medium-sized pineapple cubes to add to the salad. Now chop the aromas: chives and mint. Take the mixed salad previously washed under water and pour it into the pineapple container along with its cubes. Also, add the previously sautéed prawns. Then add the aromatic herbs to the salad: chives, minced mint salt, a drizzle of oil, and mix the ingredients to blend the flavors.

Now that the salad is ready, you can start stuffing the pineapple until it is full. Now you can serve your pineapple shrimp salad for a beautiful and fresh summer lunch!

4) Chickpea shrimp and arugula salad

Ingredients:

- Shrimp 1 kg
- Pre-cooked chickpeas 240 g
- Rocket 150 g
- Pine nuts 30 g
- **TO CONDITION**

- **Lemon juice 1**
- **Extra virgin olive oil to taste**
- **Salt to taste**

To make the chickpea shrimp and rocket salad, start by cleaning the shrimp (or prawns) by removing the head, the carapace, and the intestines inside. Now toast the pine nuts in a pan for 4-5 minutes until they are browned and set aside. Heat a drizzle of oil in a pan, put the prawns, salt, use a pinch of pepper. Cook them on high heat for 5 -6 minutes. Once cooked, transfer them to a small bowl to cool. Now drain the pre-cooked chickpeas (you can also use the dried ones but keep them soak and cook them for at least three hours so they will be ready for preparation). In the same pan used for the prawns, heat the chickpeas so that they take on the flavor of the shellfish.

Now that all the ingredients are ready, you can compose the salad: In a large bowl, put the washed and dried arugula. Add the prawns, chickpeas and toasted pine nuts and mix everything together. Finally, take care of the dressing: prepare an emulsion with oil, salt, and the juice of half a lemon. Season the salad with the prepared dressing. Your chickpea shrimp and rocket salad are now ready!

5) Vegetable crudités

Ingredients:

- **Celery 2**
- **Carrots 2**
- **Fennel 1**
- **Yellow peppers 1/2**
- **1/2 red peppers**
- **Chicory 1**
- **Radishes 12**
- **Extra virgin olive oil to taste**
- **Lemon juice to taste**
- **Salt to taste**

Take two stalks of tender celery and clean them by removing the leaves and any filaments. Cut the stalks into two parts of equal length and then cut the sticks by cutting the pieces obtained for the length. Take the fennel, remove the ends with the leaves, and then also the opposite one; now cut the fennel into four equal parts, which you will reduce again in half. Take the half peppers, remove the filaments and the internal white parts, then cut the peppers into strips. Remove the radish leaves and wash the radishes under running water. Peel the carrots, tick the ends, and cut them into parallel slices, which you will then divide into sticks. Remove the outer leaves of the radicchio and keep them fresh and intact by detaching them from its base.

Now put the vegetables cut into small glasses and prepare bowls containing extra virgin olive oil. To prepare the sauce, mix together in a salt oil container, lemon, and beat vigorously with a fork to emulsify everything or do it with an immersion blender. Serve your vegetable sticks accompanied by the sauce.

6) Chunks of quinoa

Ingredients:

- **Quinoa 150 g**
- **Small zucchini 2**
- **Eggs 1**
- **Grated cheese 50 g**
- **Grated lemon zest 1**
- **Fresh ginger to be grated to taste**
- **Salt to taste**

Proceed by draining the quinoa and passing it under cold water to stop cooking. At this point, wash the zucchini and peel them, then peel and peel the fresh ginger. Grate the zucchini and place them in a large bowl, where you will add the grated fresh ginger and the grated lemon zest. Add the boiled quinoa to the grated zucchini, ginger, and lemon zest and add the grated cheese and egg. Season with salt and mix the ingredients until you obtain a homogeneous mixture. Now put the mixture in baking molds (you can also use a non-stick muffin mold) and place them on a baking sheet. Compact the mixture inside the shapes with the help of the back of a spoon, in order to better define the shape of the morsels. Now bake them in an oven already preheated in static mode at 180 ° for 25 minutes (if you use a fan oven cook them at 160 ° for 20 minutes), until the surface is golden brown. At this point, the quinoa morsels are ready to be tasted!

7) Eggplant Caviar

Ingredients:

- **Eggplant (about 3) 1 kg**
- **½ lemon juice**
- **Mint 4 leaves**
- **Extra virgin olive oil 2 tbsp**
- **Salt to taste**

Wash the eggplant, then dry them. Arrange them on a dripping pan lined with a sheet of parchment paper. Cook them in a preheated static oven at 180 ° for at least 60 minutes (or at 160 ° for 50 minutes if in a fan oven).

Now remove the eggplants from the oven, and with a knife, remove the peel and with a spoon take the pulp contained inside. Put the pulp in a narrow mesh strainer and with the back of a spoon press it, so that it releases the excess liquid. Put the pulp in a mixer equipped with blades and add the oil.

Season with salt and add the mint after which operate the blades until you get a thick and homogeneous puree. Transfer everything to a small bowl, then squeeze the juice of half a lemon into the puree you have obtained. Mix everything, and your eggplant caviar is ready to be served.

8) Octopus salad

Ingredients:

- **Octopus to clean 1 kg**
- **Carrots 1**
- **Celery 1 rib**
- **Laurel 2 leaves**
- **Salt up to 4 g**

TO CONDITION
- **Parsley 10 g**
- **Lemon juice 10 g**
- **Extra virgin olive oil 30 g**
- **Black pepper 1 pinch**
- **Salt up to a pinch**

Start with the octopus, rinse it under running water, with a knife cut the bag at eye level to eliminate them, then also remove the beak. Rinse the octopus again under running water and remove the entrails from the bag by washing it carefully inside (You can also use the frozen one). Peel the carrot, then cut it into coarse pieces. Do the same thing with celery. Place a large saucepan with water on the fire, pour the coast of celery into pieces, the pieces of carrot, the bay leaves, and add the salt.

When the water has touched the boil, dip the octopus in the pan and cook over very low heat for 40-45 minutes, covering with a lid. As it cooks, you can remove residues and foam that are created on the surface from the water. At the end of the cooking, let the octopus cool in the same water so that it is soft. Transfer it to the cutting board and, with a knife, separate the head from the tentacles and divide them in half. Cut the tentacles into small pieces. Cut the head into small pieces and pour everything into a bowl. For the dressing, squeeze the lemon, then wash and finely chop the parsley. Make the dressing by pouring the juice, parsley, lemon juice, oil, and salt into a jar. Close and mix. Pour the mixture over the octopus, mix well, and serve your octopus salad!

9) Marinated anchovies

Ingredients:

- **Anchovies (chopped) 500 g**
- **Lemon juice 150 g**
- **Parsley 20 g**
- **Extra virgin olive oil 140 g**
- **Fine salt**

To prepare the marinated anchovies started with the marinade: pour the parsley together with 40 g of olive oil in a mixer and chop everything for a few moments. Squeeze the lemons, and collect the juice in a container together with the olive oil and season with salt. Mix well and when the two compounds have bonded together, add the chopped parsley. Keep stirring and keep the marinade aside. Meanwhile, move on to cleaning the anchovies; given that they will not undergo cooking, it is important to make sure that they were cut down during the purchase phase (always choose fresh anchovies to buy in your trusted fish shop); for greater safety, it is recommended to freeze for at least 96 hours at -18 degrees (already gutted) and then thaw to use in the recipe. Then take off the head, then pull away the central bone and the entrails, finally rinse the fillets underwater, taking care not to divide the fish into two halves.

Place the well-cleaned anchovy fillets side by side in a large container and pour the marinade you have prepared, then cover with plastic wrap. Let stand for at least 5 hours at room temperature. After the necessary time, remove the film, and finally drain them slightly from the marinade and arrange the marinated anchovies on a plate to serve and enjoy them as an appetizer!

10) Eggplant and tofu meatballs

Ingredients:
- **100 g of tofu**
- **1 large eggplant**
- **1 clove of garlic**
- **2 sprigs of parsley**
- **1 tablespoon of flour**
- **4 tablespoons of breadcrumbs**
- **salt**
- **oil to taste**

Cook the whole eggplant in the oven; once cooked, sauté its pulp in a pan in a garlic sauce. Season with salt and add the crumbled tofu. Mix the ingredients, if necessary, with a little flour. Complete the preparation with chopped parsley. Prepare meatballs the size of an apricot, dip them in breadcrumbs, bake them or fry them in a pan, according to preference.

Chapter 5: First dishes

1) Risotto with chickpeas

Ingredients:

- **140 grams of brown rice**
- **200 grams of boiled chickpeas**
- **1 carrot**
- **1 teaspoon of extra virgin olive oil**
- **vegetable broth**

Sauté the carrot cut into small pieces with the oil in a pan. Mix and combine 150 grams of boiled chickpeas, giving flavor to everything. Add the rice and continue cooking for 15 minutes or as long as the packaging. Occasionally pour a ladle of vegetable rice broth if you see that the bottom of the pan is dry and without liquid. Cook the rice completely, and at the end of the cooking, add the remaining chickpeas. Your risotto is ready to be eaten!

2) Barley and bean soup

Ingredients:
- 200 g of cooked beans
- 150 g of pearl barley
- 1 small carrot
- 1 stalk of celery
- 100 g approx. of pumpkin pulp
- 1 sprig of parsley
- 1 clove of garlic
- 4 tablespoons of oil
- 1 pinch of chilli
- salt

Boil the barley in 400 ml of water with a pinch of salt, for about 40 minutes, in a covered pot. Prepare a mixture of garlic, celery, carrot, and parsley; cut the pumpkin into cubes. Fry the mixture in oil in a large pot with a pinch of salt; then add the pumpkin and let it simmer for five minutes, until softened, possibly with a little water. Then add the barley and beans with their cooking water or a little broth to get the right consistency (the soup should be creamy); bring to a boil and cook for another 5 minutes. Season with a pinch of chili and serve hot. Alternatively, you can cook the barley directly with the vegetables and add the beans towards cooking.

3) Pasta and zucchini

Ingredients:

- Pasta 320 g
- Zucchini 650 g
- Basil to taste
- Salt to taste
- Extra virgin olive oil 20 g
- Black pepper to taste
- Garlic 1 clove

To prepare pasta and zucchini, boil the water in a large saucepan and salt when it has come to a boil. In the meantime, wash and dry the zucchini, cut them into cubes or slices. In a large enough pan, pour the extra virgin olive oil and heat it over low heat together with a whole clove of garlic already peeled.

As soon as the oil is hot, add the zucchini, add salt and pepper and cook for 5-6 minutes, stirring occasionally, then remove the garlic. In the meantime, boil the pasta in boiling salted water and drain it al dente, keeping some cooking water aside.

Pour the pasta into the pan with the zucchini, together with a little cooking water, sauté the pasta, stir and then turn off. Perfume everything with a little chopped basil by hand, and your pasta and zucchini are ready to be enjoyed. Before bringing to the table, remove the bay leaves and possibly also the cloves and serve hot.

4) Cream of spinach with pine nuts

Ingredients:
- 1 kg of spinach
- 2 shallots
- 500 ml of vegetable broth
- 100 ml of soy milk
- 100 g of tofu
- 2 tablespoons of flour
- 2 tablespoons of pine nuts
- 2 teaspoons of turmeric
- 2 tablespoons of oil
- salt and pepper

Clean the spinach, wash and drain them. Finely chop the shallots and let them soften in a saucepan with a little broth for about ten minutes. Add the flour, stir so that it does not form lumps, and add the spinach. Add salt, stir briefly and pour in the warmed milk and remaining broth, tofu, and turmeric. Cook for about ten minutes and blend by immersion. Peppered, seasoned with oil, and served garnished with lightly toasted pine nuts and, if desired, with oatcakes

5) Indian rice

Ingredients:
- 300 g of wholemeal basmati rice
- 1 carrot
- 200 g of peas
- 2 shallots
- 1 piece of cinnamon
- 2 cardamom capsules
- 1 heaped teaspoon of turmeric
- 1 clove
- 1 bay leaf
- 1 tablespoon of raisins
- 20 almonds
- 3 tablespoons of oil
- salt and pepper

Put the rice in a saucepan, cover it with 800 ml of water, close with the lid, and boil. Turn down the heat. Rinse the raisins and soak them in warm water for about ten minutes. Put the chopped shallots in a pan with the cinnamon, the cardamom seeds, the turmeric, the clove, and the bay leaf. Add the soaking water from the raisins and let it soften over medium heat, stirring often. Transfer to the saucepan with the rice. When 30 minutes have passed, add the peas, raisins, and carrot cut into cubes. Cook for another 15-20 minutes until the liquid has run out. Remove the bay leaf, the carnation, and the cinnamon. Season with salt, season with oil and pepper. Complete with the sliced almonds and serve.

6) Rice and zucchini croquettes with saffron sauce

Ingredients:
For the croquettes:
- 350 g of brown rice
- 850 ml of water
- 800 g of zucchini
- 2 tablespoons of oil
- 1 teaspoon of salt
- 1 bunch of parsley
- 1 clove of garlic
- salt and pepper

For the saffron sauce:
- 250 ml of soy milk
- 30 ml of oil
- 30 g of rice flour
- 1 sachet of saffron and salt

Sauté the chopped garlic and parsley in a little oil. Add and stew the sliced zucchini with salt and pepper for 10 minutes. Puree about 1/3 of the zucchini. Wash the rice, drain it and cook it in salted water, covered and without stirring, for about 35 minutes. Season the rice with the salt and the zucchini not passed, stir and continue cooking for another 5 minutes.

Let it cool (if it is too soft, let it cool completely or add some breadcrumbs), then form some meatballs that you will bake in the oven at 200 ° for about 15-20 minutes. To prepare the sauce, brown the flour in a saucepan with the oil, then add the milk. Bring to a boil and let it thicken over low heat, stirring with a whisk. Salt and add the saffron and the zucchini puree.

7) Broccoli and sweet potato pie

Ingredients:
- 300 g of sweet potatoes
- 400 g of broccoli
- 2 cloves of garlic
- 1 bunch of parsley
- 1 glass of vegetable broth
- 3 tablespoons of oil
- salt

Peel and wash the sweet potatoes, then cut them into slices that are not too thick. Peel and clean the broccoli; slice the stems and divide the flowers into florets. Finely chop garlic and parsley. Line a baking sheet with parchment paper and brush it with a tablespoon of oil mixed with water. Make the first layer with the potatoes and a pinch of salt, a second with the broccoli and a little more salt, a third with garlic and parsley. Finish with the potatoes and pour over all the broth. Bake at 190 degrees for about 40 minutes. When cooked, season with the remaining oil and serve.

8) Spelled and leek lasagna

Ingredients:
- **300 g of lasagne**
- **2 leeks**
- **250 g of mozzarella**
- **70 g of parmesan cheese**
- **extra virgin olive oil**
- **½ glass of milk**

Clean the leeks, cut them lengthwise, and soak them in freshwater for about 30 minutes. Meanwhile, in a full pot of boiling water, cook the lasagna for about 5 minutes and set it aside. Drain the leeks and put them to stew in a pan with a drizzle of oil without adding salt because they are already delicious. Cook them for about twenty minutes. Take a pan, preferably rectangular, and form the layers: start by placing a layer of pasta on the pan's bottom and lay the leeks on top. Take the mozzarella, cut it into small pieces, and put them on top of the leeks. Finish with a sprinkling of parmesan cheese. Continue to alternate puff pastry, leek, mozzarella, and parmesan, until all the ingredients are used up. Once the last sheet is finished, pour the milk over the lasagna and complete it with a shower of parmesan cheese. Bake for 25 minutes at 180 °.

9) Spaghetti in tofu cream with spinach and hazelnuts

Ingredients:
- 350 g of wholemeal spaghetti
- 200 g of fresh spinach
- 80 g of hazelnuts

For the olive tofu cream
- 200 g of natural tofu
- the juice of half a lemon
- 1 cup of capers
- 1 cup of olives
- a large tuft of chopped parsley
- 3 tablespoons of olive oil
- a tablespoon of soy sauce
- a pinch of salt
- 1 small clove of garlic

Put the water on the fire to cook the pasta; once it reaches a boil, add salt and throw the wholemeal spaghetti. In the meantime, take a saucepan with a little water and put it on the stove: as soon as it boils, add a pinch of salt and dip the natural tofu block cut into small pieces. Boil for a minute, drain, and put it in the blender, where you will add the olives without the stones, the sprig of parsley, the capers, the juice of half a lemon, the clove of garlic, the oil, the soy sauce, and the pinch of salt. To soften, you can add a few tablespoons of the tofu boiling water.

Blend until you get a soft and homogeneous cream that you will keep aside. Then wash the fresh spinach leaves; you can roughly cut them or leave them whole. Dry them and keep them aside. Then take a non-stick pan and toast the hazelnuts, coarsely chopped. Drain the pasta and put it in a large bowl, and add the tofu cream to the olives; if necessary, help yourself with a little tofu cooking water, as above. Add the fresh spinach leaves, toasted hazelnuts, and finally a drizzle of raw oil. If you wish, you can also add a splash of fresh oregano or paprika powder. Serve the spaghetti hot and steaming. Simple and tasty!

10) Rice cake

Ingredients:

- **Champignon mushrooms 500 g**
- **Rice 300 g**
- **Grated cheese 150 g**
- **Vegetable broth about 750 ml**
- **1 sprig parsley**
- **Salt to taste**

Dedicate yourself to the champignon mushrooms, wash and peel them, then remove the part of the stem with the roots and cut the head of the champignons into rather thin slices. Chop the fresh parsley. In a large pan pour a drizzle of oil then add the champignon mushrooms and chopped parsley. Fry over low heat for about 3 minutes. Stir and cook the mushrooms for about 5 minutes. Season with salt and then cook for about 10 minutes over moderate heat. The mushrooms will not have to cook completely because they will then finish cooking in the oven. While the mushrooms are cooking, pour the oil into a large pan, pour in the rice, brown for a couple of minutes, stirring with a wooden spoon.

Continue cooking the risotto for about 20 minutes, adding the vegetable broth a little at a time with a ladle when you see that the rice is devoid of liquid. When the rice is cooked for 2 minutes, pour in the grated cheese, stir, turn off the heat and let the risotto rest for a few minutes. Take a baking tray and cover it with parchment paper. Then with a spoon start creating a layer of rice, compacting it with the back of the spoon. When you have covered the bottom, create a layer of mushrooms, then rice, so that the result is two layers with the mushroom filling. Finally, sprinkle the top with the leftover cheese. Finally bake in a preheated static oven at 200 ° for about 30 minutes (if oven at 180 ° for about 25 minutes). Then remove from the oven and let it cool.

Chapter 6: Main courses

1) Veal roast, apples and potatoes

Ingredients:

- 600 grams of veal fillet
- 1 teaspoon of oil
- 2 sprigs of rosemary
- half a glass of white wine
- 2 apples
- 250 grams of potatoes
- Salt

Put the meat in a pan with oil, rosemary, and a pinch of salt. Brown it by blending with the white wine. Combine the apples with the peel and the chopped potatoes. Bake at 200 degrees for about 30 minutes. Get out of the oven, remove the meat, and let it cool. Cut it into slices and serve with potatoes and apples.

2) Poached eggs

Ingredients:

- **Very fresh, organic eggs 4**
- **Coarse salt to taste**
- **White wine vinegar 10 g**
- **TO ACCOMPANY**
- **4 slices bread**

When the salt has dissolved, and the water starts to boil lightly (it must not boil strongly), lower the flame and with a whisk stir always in the same direction to create a vortex in the water; then break an egg into a small bowl and pour it in the center of the vortex. Cook the egg like this for 2 minutes. Do not mix or move the egg. Drain the egg with the help of a slotted spoon, then lay it on the toasted bread and serve your hot poached eggs.

3) Crispy salmon

Ingredients:
- Salmon fillet (4 of 250 g each) 1 kg
- Bread 100 g
- 1 sprig parsley
- Thyme 4 sprigs
- Rosemary 2 sprigs
- Lemon zest 1
- Extra virgin olive oil 50 g
- White pepper in grains 1 tsp
- Salt up to taste

First, prepare the breading: cut the bread into pieces and put it in a mixer, the peeled thyme, the needles of rosemary and parsley. Pour in the oil too, then add the lemon zest, salt and white pepper. Blend until you get a coarse consistency. Now take care of the salmon fillets: remove the skin with a thin-bladed knife and remove the bones with the help of a kitchen tongs, then transfer the fillets to a drip pan lined with parchment paper and cover them with the breading, making it adhere well with your hands. . After covering the fillets evenly, cook in a preheated convection oven at 190 ° for about 20 minutes. After the cooking time, take out and serve your crispy salmon hot!

4) Sea bass with herb in salt crust

Ingredients:

- Salt up to 1 kg
- Sea bass 800 g
- Coarse salt 1 kg
- Sage 6 leaves
- Thyme 6 sprigs
- Parsley 1 bunch
- Laurel 4 leaves
- Rosemary 3 sprigs
- Garlic 1 clove
- Lemons 1

Spread a sheet of parchment paper on a baking sheet and then lay a thin layer (about 1.5 cm) of the mixture obtained, which will form the cooking bed for the sea bass. Now place the sea bass on the bed of salt that you previously flavored by placing it in your belly aromatic herbs, minced garlic, and lemon zest; now cover the sea bass with the salt mixture by pressing it gently to make the dough adhere well and give a shape that adheres to the fish 11. Bake for about 40 minutes (if instead of 1-kilo sea bass, you have taken a smaller one 400 / About 500gr the cooking time will be about 25-30 minutes).

After 40 minutes, remove the sea bass from the oven, let it rest for a few moments, then, using a small hammer, break the salt crust and proceed to remove the skin of the fish. Open it in two by removing the central bone, as in any other oven preparation. You can accompany the sea bass, with boiled potatoes, or also cooked in the oven. Season with a drizzle of extra virgin olive oil, not to cover the aroma and delicate flavor of the sea bass.

5) Chicken and zucchini salad

Ingredients:

- Sliced chicken breast 400 g
- Zucchini 200 g
- Eggplants 200 g
- Mixed salad 60 g
- Salt to taste
- Extra virgin olive oil to taste
-

FOR MARINATING

- **Extra virgin olive oil 25 g**
- **Wildflower honey 25 g**
- **½ lemon juice**
- **Thyme to taste**
- **Salt to taste**

To prepare the chicken and zucchini salad, we must first marinate the chicken. Arrange the chicken breasts in an ovenproof dish, pour the oil inside, season with salt, the juice of half a lemon, honey, and a few sprigs of thyme. Turn the slices over both so that the entire surface of the meat is well marinated, then cover the baking dish with plastic wrap and let it sit for one hour at room temperature. Now move on to the preparation of the vegetables. Wash the zucchini, cut the ends, and cut them lengthwise with a sliced knife about 1 cm thick. Do the same thing with eggplants too. Now heat the grill, grease it with a drizzle of oil, then lay the slices of zucchini and grill them on both sides, then salt. Also, grill and salt the eggplants, turning them on both sides, then switch to the chicken, which you will pick from the marinade to put it on the grill. Once grilled, cut the eggplants, zucchini, and chicken slices into strips about 2 cm long. Let the grilled vegetables cool, and transfer them to a bowl with the chicken and the mixed salad, then mix and transfer to the dishes. The chicken and zucchini salad are ready to be served!

6) Pan-fried sea bream

Ingredients:

- **Sea bream (2 pieces) 1100 g**
- **Extra virgin olive oil 30 g**
- **Carrots 150 g**
- **Zucchini 150 g**
- **Garlic 1 clove**
- **Thyme to taste**

To prepare the sea bream in a pan, first of all, you have to clean the fish (otherwise you can buy it already gutted). Make a cut on the belly with scissors and remove the entrails with your hands, then rinse the inside thoroughly under water and eliminate the scales using a blade of a knife; do this under running water so as not to spread the scales around. Now let's cut the vegetables: wash and peel the carrots, then cut the ends and cut them into rounds. Wash and peel the courgettes and cut them into cubes.

Pour the oil into a large non-stick pan, add a clove of poached garlic and fry it for a couple of minutes. When the oil is flavored, remove the garlic from the pan and lay the sea bream inside, then add the zucchini, carrots, and thyme sprigs and salt to taste. Cover the pan with a lid and cook over medium heat for 7 minutes, then turn the sea bream with the help of 2 spatulas being careful not to break them; cover again with the lid and cook for another 7 minutes. Cooking times may vary depending on the weight of the sea bream you will use. Pan-fried sea bream is ready to eat!

7) Cod medallions and broccoli

Ingredients:

- **Cod fillet 400 g**
- **Broccoli 200 g**
- **Potatoes 400 g**
- **Marjoram 3 sprigs**
- **Extra virgin olive oil to taste**
- **Salt to taste**

To prepare the medallions of cod and broccoli, first, we take the cod fillets (they should also be frozen well, in that case, let them thaw for at least 2-3 hours before). Then put two saucepans on the fire with water to bring to a boil; in one dip the potatoes, calculate them 30-40 minutes. The time may vary depending on the size of the potatoes, so remember to check the degree of cooking with a fork. If the fork easily penetrates inside the potatoes, it means it is cooked. In the meantime, wash the broccoli, put them in the other pan, and when the water boils boil them for about 5 minutes. After 5 minutes, drain the broccoli and coarsely chop them, then let them cool. When the potatoes are ready, peel and mash them with a potato masher in a large bowl, then preheat the oven to 200 ° in static mode. Finally, take the cod fillets and cut them into several, not too small parts. When the vegetables have cooled, take the bowl where you have mashed the potatoes, add the chopped broccoli and cod, salt and add the marjoram leaves, then knead with your hands to mix all the ingredients. Take some dough and shape it with a pastry cutter to form the medallions. Place the medallions on a dripping pan lined with parchment paper, season with a little oil, then cook in a preheated static oven at 200 ° for about 20 minutes. After the cooking time of the medallions, take them out of the oven and transfer them to a serving dish; add a few leaves of marjoram and season with a drizzle of raw oil. Your cod and broccoli medallions are ready to be brought to the table!

8) Baked chicken legs

Ingredients:

- **Chicken legs 4**
- **Potatoes 500 g**
- **Salt to taste**
- **Extra virgin olive oil 50 g**
- **Rosemary 3 sprigs**
- **Thyme 3 sprigs**

Put the chicken legs in a baking dish and season with salt, oil, and marinate. Peel the potatoes, cut them into wedges, and transfer them into a dripping pan lined with parchment paper. Season with salt, oil (optional pepper but do not overdo it), then add the chicken legs and flavor everything with the sprigs of thyme and rosemary. Bake in a preheated static oven at 180 ° for 80 minutes, turning them halfway through cooking. When they are golden brown, take them out of the oven and serve them!

9) Roasted rabbit

Ingredients:

- **Rabbit in pieces 1.2 kg**
- **4 sprigs rosemary**
- **Salt to taste**
- **Vegetable broth 150 g**
- **Potatoes 800 g**
- **Thyme 4 sprigs**
- **White wine 40 g**
- **Bay leaf 1 leaf**
- **Extra virgin olive oil 70 g**

To prepare the rabbit in the oven, start by preparing the vegetable broth a couple of hours before, chop the rosemary, then transfer half of it to a pan where you have poured 40 g of oil. Add a bay leaf and let it cook over low heat for 2-3 minutes. At this point, raise the heat and add the rabbit pieces, brown them on both sides for 3-4 minutes, add salt and deglaze with the white wine. Once the alcoholic phase has evaporated, add a ladle of broth and cook over low heat for another 5-6 minutes.

Meanwhile, prepare the potatoes, peel them, cut them into large enough pieces, and transfer them to a bowl. Add chopped rosemary, thyme leaves and salt to the potatoes. Sprinkle with 20 g of oil and mix. Transfer everything to a large pan, oiled with about 10 g of oil. Then arrange the browned rabbit pieces as well. Add the remaining vegetable broth and cook the rabbit together with the potatoes in a preheated static oven at 200 ° for 40 minutes. Once cooked, serve your rabbit in the oven

10) Salad baskets with turkey

Ingredients:
- **Turkey breast 250 g**
- **Baby lettuce 100 g**
- **Cashews 25 g**
- **Carrots 1**
- **Parsley to taste**
- **Extra virgin olive oil q.s.**

Place the turkey breast on a cutting board and cut it into irregular pieces. Then take a non-stick pan, heat a drizzle of oil. Add the turkey breast bites and salt. Cook the morsels for about 10 minutes, turning them from time to time to cook them inside until they are golden brown. When the turkey morsels are cooked, transfer them to a mixer, operate for a few seconds until the meat is well chopped, and then transfer the blended mixture into a large bowl. At this point, place the cashews on a cutting board and chop them coarsely. Sauté the chopped cashews in a non-stick pan and toast them for a few minutes, until crisp and darker. Then add the toasted cashews to the chopped turkey bites. Then take a carrot, peel it and divide it in half. After that, slice it into tiny cubes.

Also, wash the parsley under running water and chop finely on a cutting board. At this point, add the diced carrot and chopped parsley to the mixture. Now wash the salad carefully and leaf it through, placing the crispest and most curved leaves on a serving dish. Then proceed to fill them with the dough. Your baskets of lettuce with turkey are ready to be served.

Chapter 7: Recipes for Side dish

1) Fennel in a pan

Ingredients:

- Fennel (about 2) 900 g
- Extra virgin olive oil 15 g
- Himalayan salt (pink) to taste
- Marjoram to taste
- Thyme to taste

To make the fennel in a pan, start by washing the fennel, then clean them by cutting the base of the core, and the stalks, after which cut them into wedges. Once the fennel is cut, you can proceed with cooking: heat the extra virgin olive oil in a pan, then add the fennel wedges and cook for about 5 minutes on high heat. Season with the Himalayan salt and season with the leaves of marjoram and thyme. Continue cooking for another 5 minutes to keep the fennel crunchy otherwise, and you can continue cooking them for a few more minutes if you like them softer. Serve your fennel hot in a pan.

2) Carrot and sweet potato roll with millet

Ingredients:
- 200 g of carrots
- 1 sweet potato
- 1 tablespoon of corn starch
- 200 g of cooked millet
- 3 tablespoons of oil
- salt

To garnish
- 100 g of peeled pumpkin
- a few leaves of salad
- 1 tablespoon of oil
- salt

Clean the carrots and the potato, chop them and steam them for about 10 minutes. Let them cool, then blend them in the mixer with the millet, starch, oil, and salt. Remove the salami mixture and wrap it in cotton gauze, closing them like candy with a piece of string. Steam them for 15-20 minutes. Wait until they are completely cold and cut them into slices. Wash the salad, dry it and cut it into strips; coarsely grate the pumpkin. Arrange the rolls on a serving dish, surround them with the prepared garnish seasoned with oil and salt.

3) Grilled vegetables

Ingredients:

- **Zucchini 300 g**
- **Eggplants 450 g**
- **Peppers 850 g**
- **Salt to taste**

To prepare the grilled vegetables, wash all the vegetables under running fresh water, and dry them. Cut the zucchini and eggplants into slices; take the peppers, remove the upper part, divide them in half, and with a knife remove the white filaments and the seeds that are inside. Cut them into rather large cubes and set aside. Cut all the vegetables, heat the grill.

When the grill is hot, cook the vegetables a little at a time. Spread the peppers close to each other, grilling them for 5 minutes and turning them over for even cooking, then put the eggplants on the fire for 3 minutes and continue with the zucchini for another 3 minutes. Remember to always turn the vegetables over for even cooking. Finally, season the grilled vegetables with olive oil and salt.

4) Mashed potatoes

Ingredients:

- **Yellow potatoes 1 kg**

- **Whole skimmed 200 g**

- **Light butter 30 g**

- **Parmigiano Reggiano to be grated 30 g**

- **Salt to taste**

- **Nutmeg to taste**

Let's start by boiling the potatoes. Then pour them in a large pot and cover with plenty of water. Put the pan on the fire, and when the water has boiled, it will take 40 to 50 minutes. The cooking times depend on the size of the potatoes. Reached the 40 minutes of cooking skewer a potato with a fork and see if it penetrates easily; at that point, it is cooked. Drain and let it cool for a few minutes because you will have to take advantage that the potatoes are still very hot to peel them easily.

After peeling the potatoes, pour them into the potato masher, pour them directly into the cooking pan. Then add a pinch of salt and flavor by grating a little nutmeg. In the meantime, put the milk in a saucepan.
Meanwhile, light over a low flame where there is a pot with the mashed potatoes, and when the milk is hot, pour it inside and mix with a whisk until the mixture is well blended. Then turn off the heat and stir adding butter and Parmesan cheese. Your mashed potato is read.

5) Baked au gratin vegetables

Ingredients:

- Zucchini 300 g
- Eggplants 180 g long
- Red peppers 250 g
- Yellow peppers 250 g
- Extra virgin olive oil 20 g
- Salt to taste

FOR BREADING

- Breadcrumbs 30 g
- Parmesan cheese DOP to be grated 30 g
- Dried oregano to taste

First, cut the vegetables: wash the eggplants, remove the ends, and cut them diagonally into slices 2-3 cm thick; do the same thing with the zucchini. Finally, wash the peppers, empty them of the seeds and internal filaments and cut them first in half and then into pieces more or less as big as the slices of eggplants and zucchini.

Arrange the cut vegetables in a pan lined with parchment paper, then season with salt and olive oil 6. Bake the pan in a static preheated oven at 180 ° for 45 minutes. In the meantime, prepare the breadcrumbs for the vegetables: In a bowl, add the breadcrumbs with the grated Parmesan and the oregano, and mix well. After 45 minutes, remove the vegetables from the oven, spread the breadcrumbs over all the vegetables with a spoon. Bake at 180 ° again for another 15 minutes. Your side dish is ready!

6) Artichoke salad

Ingredients:

- **Artichokes (about 6) 1 kg**
- **Lemons for acidulated water 1**

FOR THE CITRONETTE

- **Lemon juice 30 g**
- **Salt to taste**
- **Black pepper to taste**
- **Extra virgin olive oil 60**

Start by cleaning the artichokes: prepare the acidulated water to store the artichokes without oxidizing them as you clean them. Fill a bowl with water and squeeze the juice of 1 lemon inside. Remove part of the stem of the artichokes and the more leathery leaves. With a knife cut off the tip and the outermost part of the stem to keep the inside tender. Clean the artichoke, divide it into two equal parts, thinly slice the artichokes, and place them in the bowl with acidified water as you cut them. Once the cleaning is finished, put them to drain in a colander. In the meantime, take care of the seasoning.

Squeeze 30 g of lemon juice and add it to 60 g of olive oil, salt and mix the emulsion with a whisk. Pour the artichokes into a bowl and flavor them with the citronette, mix and then serve the salad on the serving dishes!

7) Breadcumb Potatoes

Ingredients:

- **Potatoes 1 kg**
- **2 sprigs rosemary**
- **Bread crumbs 50 g**
- **Sage 3 leaves**
- **Extra virgin olive oil to taste**
- **Salt to taste**

Peel the potatoes and cut them into wedges, then place them in a bowl with water so as not to blacken them. Meanwhile, finely chop the sage, rosemary, and set aside. Now take the breadcrumbs and the chopped herbs. Now drain the potato wedges with a strainer and pour the chopped breadcrumbs and season with a drizzle of olive oil and salt.

Stir and pour into a baking tray lined with parchment paper and cover the potatoes with a spoonful of breadcrumbs. Bake the potatoes in a static oven at 180 ° for 40 minutes (if the oven is at 160 ° for 30 minutes). When cooked, your potatoes will be golden and crispy, take them out of the oven and let them cool before serving.

8) Crunchy salad

Ingredients:

- **Iceberg salad 1 large head**
- **Parmigiano Reggiano one piece or in flakes 80 g**
- **Carrots 2**
- **4 slices sandwich bread**
- **Chopped parsley 3 tbsp**
- **Anchovies fillets 8**
- **Lemon juice**
- **Salt to taste**
- **Extra virgin olive oil 2 tablespoons for frying, plus q.s. to season**

Wash the iceberg salad leaves, cut them finely, and put them in a large salad bowl. Now pass the carrots and with a potato peeler cut the carrots finely with a potato peeler; always with the potato peeler, do the same also with the Parmesan cheese. Chop the anchovy fillets and parsley and place them in a bowl with oil, salt and mix everything with a fork and leave them for a few minutes to rest. Take the slices of sandwich bread, remove the darker edges, and cut them into 1 cm cubes on each side.

In a pan, add two tablespoons of extra virgin olive oil, heat it and then throw it into the cubes of bread over moderate heat, turning them on all sides. Once golden, place them on absorbent kitchen paper 11. Add the carrots, Parmesan, and the oil and parsley dressing to the iceberg salad. Mix the ingredients and then add the crispy croutons 15. Ready-made salad!

9) Ginger gourd

Ingredients:

- **Pumpkin 1 kg**
- **Fresh ginger 40 g**
- **Leeks 1**
- **Vegetable broth 500 ml**
- **Extra virgin olive oil 20 g**
- **Salt to taste**

Let's start by cleaning the pumpkin, cut it in half, empty it of the seeds and internal filaments, remove the peel, and cut it into cubes. And cut it into small cubes. Wash the leek, peel it and keep the white part of the stem that you will slice in thin slices. Place a large pan on the heat, pour the leeks and season with the olive oil and fry until the leek is wilted (about 5 minutes).

At this point, pour a ladle of hot broth and add the ginger and the pumpkin cubes and salt. Pour another ladle of broth and cook over medium heat for about 25-30 minutes, adding broth little by little during cooking so as not to dry the vegetables too much. When the pumpkin is soft, turn off the heat. The ginger pumpkin is ready to be brought to the table.

10) Roasted carrots with pistachio

Ingredients:

- **Carrots 650 g**
- **Unsalted pistachios 80 g**
- **Rosemary 3 sprigs**
- **Salt to taste**
- **Extra virgin olive oil to taste**

Wash the carrots, peel them, divide them in half and then make some sticks by cutting them for the long side. Pour the carrots into a bowl and season with rosemary, olive oil, and salt. Now roughly chop the pistachios with a knife.

Add the pistachios to the carrots and mix them to amalgamate all the ingredients. Line a baking sheet with parchment paper and pour the carrots trying to distribute them evenly in order to facilitate cooking. Bake in a preheated static oven at 220 ° for 30 minutes. Once cooked, take the roasted carrots out of the oven and let them cool before serving.

Chapter 8: Recipes for dessert

1) Cocoa pudding

Ingredients:
- 500 ml of soy milk
- 4 tablespoons of unsweetened cocoa
- 3-4 tablespoons of brown sugar
- 2 tablespoons of corn starch
- 1 pinch of natural vanilla
- 1 pinch of ground cinnamon
- chopped hazelnuts to decorate

Sift the cocoa, starch, and sugar; collect them in a saucepan together with cinnamon and vanilla. First, add 100 ml of milk, stirring well to remove all lumps, and then the rest. Over medium heat, bring to a boil without stopping stirring. Lower the heat and cook for a couple of minutes more until the mixture has thickened. Moisten four single-portion molds and pour the pudding. Let it cool down and put it in the fridge until completely cooled. Decorate with the grains and serve.

2) Baked stuffed apples

Ingredients:
- 6 apples
- 1 orange
- ¾ cup of shelled walnuts
- ¾ cup of raisins
- ¼ cup of natural apple juice
- 1 tablespoon of miso

Wash and with a knife, starting from the top of the apple, make room for the filling. Heat the oven to 150 °. Rinse the raisins and chop them with the walnuts. Wash the orange and finely grate the zest. Add the orange zest, miso, and a teaspoon to the raisin and nut mixture. Mix well. Stuff the apples with the dough. Arrange the apples in a baking dish. Pierce them with a fork all around so that they do not explode during cooking. Pour the apple and orange juice into the pan and bake in the oven for half an hour. Eat them warm or cold.

3) Spiced apple pie

Ingredients:
- 3 apples
- 200 g of spelled flour type 0
- 30 g of corn starch
- 50 g of raisins
- 50 g of peeled and chopped almonds
- 150-200 ml of almond or soy milk
- 120 ml of concentrated apple juice
- 50 ml of corn oil
- ½ teaspoon of cinnamon
- ½ teaspoon of vanilla
- 1 pinch of clove powder
- the grated zest of ½ lemon
- ½ sachet of baking powder
- 1 pinch of salt

Cut the apples into small pieces, soak the raisins. In a bowl, mix the flour, starch, almonds, spices, lemon peel, salt, and yeast; in another, milk, concentrated juice, oil, apples, and drained raisins. Mix all the ingredients, transfer the mixture into a pan lined with parchment paper and bake at 190 ° for about 45 minutes. Check the cooking with a toothpick before serving.

4) Carrot cake

Ingredients:
- **200 g of wholemeal flour**
- **80 g of almonds**
- **80 g of raisins**
- **200 g of carrots**
- **100 g of rice malt**
- **4 tablespoons of sunflower oil**
- **1 orange**
- **3 tablespoons of corn starch**
- **1 teaspoon of yeast**
- **½ teaspoon of natural vanilla**
- **soya milk**
- **1 pinch of salt**

Wash the orange, grate the zest and squeeze the juice. Put the first in a bowl together with the flour, finely ground almonds, starch, yeast, vanilla, and salt. Stir. Mix the oil, malt, and orange juice in a bowl. Gradually add them to the dry ingredients. Complete with grated carrots and rinsed raisins. If the dough is too firm, dilute it with a little soy milk. Line a square mold of about 20 cm on each side with baking paper. Transfer the mixture, level it, and bake at 180 degrees for about 45 minutes. Check the cooking with a toothpick, which must come out dry. Let the cake cool in the pan, turn it out of the mold, and let it cool.

5) Banana dessert

Ingredients:
- 50 g of pitted dates
- 10 g of sultanas
- 100 g of Pecan nuts
- 50 g of peeled almonds
- 50 g of Rapè coconut
- Himalayan salt
- 1 tablespoon of orange juice
- 1 tablespoon of coconut oil
- cinnamon powder

For the stuffing
- 2 large bananas
- 420 g of cashews soaked for about 6-7 hours
- the juice and grated zest of ½ organic lemon
- 150 ml of agave syrup, cooled in the freezer for about 25 minutes
- 150 g of cocoa butter
- 1 tablespoon of coconut oil

To garnish
- ½ bar of dark chocolate or maple syrup or chopped hazelnuts
- banana slices (optional)

Wash the dates and raisins under running water, then chop them finely in a mixer; without turning off the appliance, add the salt, orange juice, coconut oil, and cinnamon. When you have obtained a compact mixture, add the Pecan nuts and the chopped almonds in thin grains separately, complete with the Rapè coconut. Mix the dough well and roll it out on the bottom of a small cake pan (or a loaf pan), which you will have lined with baking paper. Level it well on the surface using a spatula and put it to solidify in the freezer or refrigerator.

Drain the cashews and grind them for a long time in the mixer to make them doughy. Continuing to operate, first add the lemon juice and zest, agave syrup, cocoa butter, and melted coconut oil; then add the bananas and continue until you have a soft cream. Pour it on the cooled base and place it in the freezer, so that it becomes firm. You can also divide it into individual portions. Let it cool for a few minutes before serving. Decorate with a few banana slices, if you like, or with dark chocolate cut into flakes or with maple syrup and chopped hazelnuts.

6) Almond and apricot cake

Ingredients:
- 500g of chopped apricots + other ripe ones for garnish
- ½ cup of chopped dried apricots
- 2 tablespoons of agar-agar
- 2 cups of almond milk
- 2 tablespoons of almond cream
- the grated zest of ½ lemon
- 1 teaspoon of vanilla
- 4 tablespoons of corn starch
- ½ cup of concentrated apple juice
- 200 g of ladyfingers
- Apple juice
- salt

Put the fresh and dried apricots in a pot together with half a cup of water, the agar-agar, and a pinch of salt. Stirring constantly, bring to a boil, and cook for 5-10 minutes. When cooked, add the concentrated juice, then blend. Use a little almond milk to dissolve the corn starch and rest on the heat with a pinch of salt, lemon peel, and vanilla. When it is about to boil, remove it from the stove, add the almond cream and starch, and then let it boil again and turn it off. Blend the apricots, add the cream and adjust the flavor by adding, if necessary, more concentrated apple juice.

Cut the ladyfingers at one end and quickly dip them in the apple juice. Arrange them standing along the edge of a mold of about 22 cm and distribute the cutouts on the bottom. Cover with the apricot cream and leave to cool for a few hours. Remove the hinge from the mold and serve the cake decorated with some halved fresh apricots.

7) Strawberry tartlets

Ingredients:
For the shortcrust pastry
- 250 g of wholemeal flour
- 50 g of coconut butter
- 2 tablespoons of rice flour
- 2 tablespoons of brown sugar
- 1 teaspoon of ground cinnamon
- 1 pinch of pink salt

For coverage
- 4 tablespoons of unsweetened apricot jam
- 2 tablespoons of chopped hazelnuts
- ½ tablespoon of lemon juice
- 1 tablespoon of cherry, plum or apricot distillate
- 400 g of strawberries
- 1 sprig of mint

Melt the coconut butter in a double boiler and let it cool. Pour it into the mixer with the other ingredients and sugar. Operate; when large crumbs begin to form, add a few tablespoons of cold water at a time, continuing to knead the dough until it collects into a ball. Wrap it in a cloth and put it in the fridge for 30 minutes. It is using a damp brush, grease 8 molds with a diameter of 10 cm with oil. Obtain from the thinly rolled dough as many discs large enough to cover the molds' walls and the bottom. They will have to adhere everywhere. Prick the bottom with a fork.

Cover each tart with a piece of parchment paper and a few dried beans. Bake at 180 degrees for 15 minutes, remove the paper and the legumes, cook them for another 5 minutes. After another ten minutes, remove them, and once cold, unmold them. Heat the jam with the distillate until it is shiny. Turn off and add the lemon juice. After a few minutes, brush part of the mixture on the bases. Wash the strawberries, dry them gently and slice them not too thin. Distribute them over the dough. Cover with the remaining jam, sprinkle the surface with the grains, and let it rest in a cool place for about an hour. Just before serving, garnish the tarts with mint leaves.

8) Chocolate with avocado and orange

Ingredients:
- 200 g of pitted dates soaked for 15 minutes
- 150 g of walnut kernels
- 150 g of white almonds
- 1 tablespoon of orange juice
- 1 tablespoon of coconut oil
- ½ teaspoon of sea salt

For the stuffing
- 5 large ripe avocados, peeled
- 100 g of coconut oil
- 1 tablespoon of white almond cream
- 50 g of melted cocoa butter
- the grated zest of ½ orange
- ½ teaspoon of vanilla powder
- 170 g of cocoa powder
- 250 g of agave syrup

To garnish
- dark chocolate grains

Soak the dates for 15 minutes. Let the maple syrup cool in the freezer for about 25 minutes. Finely grind the walnuts and almonds in the bowl of a mixer. Keep them aside. In their place, put the drained dates and purée them. Then, continuing to operate the appliance, add the salt, coconut oil, orange juice, and the previously prepared grains.

When you have a compact mixture, the spread is based on a pan (or a loaf pan) lined with baking paper. Level it well with a spatula and remove it in the freezer or in the refrigerator to make it firm. Gather all the ingredients required for the filling in a mixer and start. You will need to get a well blended mixture. Pour on the solidified base and pass the cake in the refrigerator or freezer so that it hardens. Decorated with one of the proposed alternatives and served.

9) Chocolate nut and almond balls

Ingredients:
- **200 g of wholemeal flour**
- **150 g of walnuts**
- **50 g of pine nuts**
- **50 g of sunflower seeds**
- **200 g of almonds**
- **50 g of flax seeds**
- **100 g of raisins**
- **100 g of dark chocolate in small pieces**
- **400 g of rice malt**
- **1 lemon**
- **1 orange**
- **6 tablespoons of brown sugar**

Soak the raisins in warm water. In the meantime, grate the peel of a lemon and an organic orange and place them in a large bowl. Add the coarsely chopped walnuts and almonds, flax seeds, sunflower seeds, and pine nuts. Stir in the flour, chocolate, and squeezed raisins and mix well with your hands. Then add the malt and continue to mix all the ingredients with energy. Lightly moisten your hands and form medium-sized balls that you will arrange quite far from each other in a baking tray lined with baking paper. Bake for about 10-12 minutes at 180 °. Let cool before serving. Excellent served accompanied by a fragrant compote of apples and spices.

10) Chocolate truffles

Ingredients:
- 100 g of dark chocolate
- 100 g of almonds
- 50 g of hazelnuts
- 100 g of dates
- 50 g of bitter cocoa

Soak the almonds in a glass jar for at least 3 hours, then add the dates and leave them for another hour. Meanwhile, heat the dark chocolate in a bain-marie. Drain and set aside the almond and date water. We combine the melted chocolate in the jar with the dried fruit and work it all with the hand blender. Incorporate the chopped hazelnuts and place them in the fridge for an hour. If the mixture is too hard, wet it with one or two tablespoons of soaking liquid. We sprinkle the cocoa on a saucer. We take small doses of the mixture and let them fall on the cocoa. We form balls and compact them well, trying to press them as much as possible. Let's put them in small bowls and skewer each ball with a wooden stick.

11) Tuna sauce

Ingredients:
- 100 g of tuna in oil
- 50 g of pickled capers
- 2 anchovies
- 1 firm yolk
- the juice of 1/2 lemon
- 1 glass of extra virgin olive oil
- salt
- pepper

To make the tuna sauce, start chopping the tuna well drained from the oil and collect it in the mixing bowl together with the rinsed and squeezed capers, the boned anchovies, and the crumbled hard-boiled egg yolk. Soften the dough with a few tablespoons of oil and operate the appliance with short interrupted clicks. Gradually add the rest of the oil and blend for a few seconds until the desired density is obtained. Add the lemon juice filtered through a colander and mix very well. Taste and, if necessary, season with salt and pepper. Let it sit for 10 minutes. If the sauce is too thick, dilute it with a little oil. Then pour the tuna sauce in a gravy boat or a serving bowl and serve.

Chapter 9: Drinks&Shakes

1) Golden milk

Ingredients:

- **Water 130 g**
- **Turmeric powder 40 g**
- **Black pepper 1 pinch**
- **FOR A GOLDEN MILK CUP**
- **Vegetable milk (almond or soy) 150 g**
- **honey 1 tbsp**

To prepare the golden milk, you have to start with turmeric paste. Pour the water in a saucepan together with a little pepper and bring to a boil. As soon as the water boils, turn off the heat and add the turmeric powder. Stir until you have a thick and grainy paste. Finally, transfer the turmeric paste to a jar in which you can store it. Now move on to the preparation of your cup of golden milk. In a saucepan, bring the vegetable milk to a boil and then transfer it to a jar and add a teaspoon of turmeric paste, then sweeten with honey and close the jar with the cap. Ready for your golden milk!

2) Banana milkshake

Ingredients:

- **Bananas 300 g**
- **Ice 60 g**
- **Cinnamon sticks 2 g**
- **Whole milk 150 g**

To prepare the banana smoothie, we start by cutting the bananas into chunks and inserting them in the mixer. Also, add the cinnamon, not too many ice cubes, and the milk at a standing temperature. Operate the mixer until a thick and creamy mixture is obtained. Then pour it into the glasses and decorate with a few pieces of cinnamon. The milkshake is ready.

3) Yogurt smoothie

Ingredients:

- **Yogurt 250 g**
- **Lime juice (about 1) 13 g**
- **Pulp melon 420**
- **Pulp peaches 350**

Let's start by washing the peaches (it will take about 3), peel them, and remove them from the core, then cut them into coarse pieces and set them aside. Now the melon: cut it in half, remove the seeds and peel and cut it into pieces. Cut the lime in half and squeeze it. Collect the juice obtained in a glass and keep it aside. Now take a blender and put the and melon. Pour the yogurt and lime juice, close the blender, and activate it. Keep blending until the mixture is creamy. Your yogurt smoothie is ready!

4) Almond milk

Ingredients:

- **Peeled almonds 200 g**
- **Water 1 l**
- **Acacia honey 85 g**

To prepare almond milk, first put the almonds in a bowl with 500 g of water for at least an hour to soak. After the hour, pour both the almonds and the water into a mixer, then add the remaining 500 g of water and honey. Blend everything until a homogeneous cream is obtained, then filter the mixture obtained through a narrow mesh strainer and refrigerate for at least an hour, covered with plastic wrap. Serve your almond milk cold or at room temperature.

5) Homemade tropical fruit juice

Ingredients:

- 450 g of pineapple
- 250g mango
- 2 oranges
- 1 grapefruit
- 1.2 liters of water
- 100g of sugar

Start by peeling the mango and cutting it into cubes. Peel the pineapple by cutting the ends first then in half and finally in four parts. Remove the central hard part and also make the cubes pineapple. After this, extract the juice of an orange and a grapefruit. Now transfer the citrus juice and fruit cubes to the pot with water and sugar and cook for 15 minutes. Pass 15 minutes with a hand blender and whisk until you have a puree, and you will put them in sterilized glass jars. Close the jars and put them and put them in the refrigerator until the jars cool down. They are now ready to be tasted!

6) Non-alcoholic melon cocktail

Ingredients:

- 1 untreated lemon
- 20 grams of sugar
- 2 slices of melon
- 2 slices of white melon
- 400 milliliters of carbonated mineral water

Rinse the lemon and peel without throwing away the zest. Divide the lemon in half, squeeze it, and filter the juice obtained by passing it in a colander. Put the filtered juice and the lemon zest in a saucepan together with 20 grams of sugar. Cook everything for 2 minutes on low heat, stirring. Filter the syrup obtained and let it cool. Peel the melon and the white melon, remove the seeds and the white filaments. Cut the pulp of the melons into small pieces. Put the melon pieces in the blender until you have obtained a homogeneous mixture. Add the previously prepared syrup to the melon smoothie. Incorporate, little by little, the carbonated mineral water to your non-alcoholic cocktail. Blend again and put them in a container or cocktail glasses and put them in the refrigerator. Leave them to cool for a quarter of an hour. When finished, decorate the glasses as desired with straws and melon slices. Serve the non-alcoholic melon cocktail still very fresh.

7) Smoothie cheesecake

Ingredients:

- **Lean cottage cheese 250 g**
- **Fresh liquid cream 250 g**
- **Icing sugar 30 g**
- **Strawberries 280 g**
- **Yellow peaches 380 g**

To make the cheesecake smoothie, first, wash the peach and strawberries, then peel the peach and cut it into pieces, transfer it to the mixer glass and blend to get a puree. Do the same operation with the strawberries, remove the green stalk, cut them into small pieces, and place in the mixer glass to blend them until you get a puree. Now pour the ricotta into a bowl, add ¾ of the fresh liquid cream, the icing sugar and blend everything with the immersion mixer to obtain a homogeneous cream. Now add the remaining fresh liquid cream and mix to mix.

Now make your own cheesecake smoothie. Use glasses of about 70 cl capacity. The smoothie is made up of a layer of ricotta cream alternated with fruit puree. Pour the first layer of cream, move the glass slightly between your hands to evenly distribute the first layer on the bottom, cover with peach or strawberry puree, then pour a layer of ricotta cream again and finish with the strawberry or peach puree. Serve your cheesecake smoothie fresh!

8) Apple cider

Ingredients:

- **700 grams of apples**
- **50 grams of sugar**
- **100 ml of water**
- **1 orange**
- **1 lemon**
- **2 cloves**
- **1 cinnamon stick**
- **1 fresh ginger**

To prepare the apple cider, start by cutting and squeezing the orange and obtaining the juice. Do the same with the lemon. Now wash, peel, and remove the core from the apples. At this point, cut the apples until they are cubed and put in the blender until the juice is obtained, then filter it with a strainer.

Now add the sugar and the orange and lemon juice and mix so as to mix all the flavors. Now add the fresh ginger, the cloves, the cinnamon, and cook for 10 minutes. Pass the 10 minutes and filter everything, and your apple cider is ready!

9) Chai latte

Ingredients:

- 200 ml milk
- 200 ml water
- 2 black tea bags
- 1 pinch of cinnamon
- 1 pinch of cardamom
- 2 ginger sticks
- 1 teaspoon maple syrup

Start by putting the water in a saucepan and bring it to a boil. Once the water boils, turn off the stove and insert the tea bags and spices. After a couple of minutes, remove the tea bags and keep them brewing for another 4 minutes.

In the meantime, take another saucepan and pour milk and a teaspoon of maple syrup. With a wooden spoon, mix well until the syrup has completely drained. You can now add the infusion in the milk and mix well to mix the flavors. Ready!

10) Fruit and yogurt cocktails

Ingredients:

- **25 gr of strawberries**
- **25 gr of raspberries**
- **125 ml of cold milk**
- **125 ml of Cold Natural Yogurt**
- **1 Teaspoon Rose Water**
- **1/2 teaspoon of light honey**

To prepare it, put the milk, strawberries, raspberries, yogurt, rose water in the blender, and blend for about 30 seconds, mixing the ingredients well. Pour into a tall drink glass, mix and add the honey. Decorate with strawberry slices or a sprig of mint, serve immediately.

Conclusion

GERD is a disorder related to the stomach and digestive system that creates irritation. The main reason behind this problem is poor nutrition, poor digestion, lack of sleep, and an incorrect lifestyle. Weight gain and other health complications can cause acid reflux. With GERD, heartburn is felt, and there is a feeling that food is coming back from the stomach. The treatments to combat GERD in the initial phase is the correct intake of food, exercise, and following a healthy diet trying to reduce weight. If not treated well, it can cause further serious health complications such as cancer or ulcers. To get quick relief from GERD, you need to adopt some lifestyle changes such as taking small meals instead of full meals, following an exercise routine, reducing, limiting the intake of spicy and fried foods, and reducing. In the initial phase of GERD, it can be treated and prevented with healthy and organic food choices. Also, carry out an adequate medical check-up; this will help you find out how serious the problem is. Consult your family doctor and listen to his or her treatment recommendations and precautions. This is the first step you need to take to treat GERD. In this book, a series of healthy and organic recipes are mentioned that will help you finally enjoy good food and relief even in acid reflux conditions.

www.ingramcontent.com/pod-product-compliance
Lightning Source LLC
Chambersburg PA
CBHW070615220526
45466CB00001B/9